Acupuncture AND Moxibustion

针灸

Traditional Chinese Medicine

PRACTICAL HANDBOOK

Sumiko Knudsen

Ph.D
Practitioner. DK

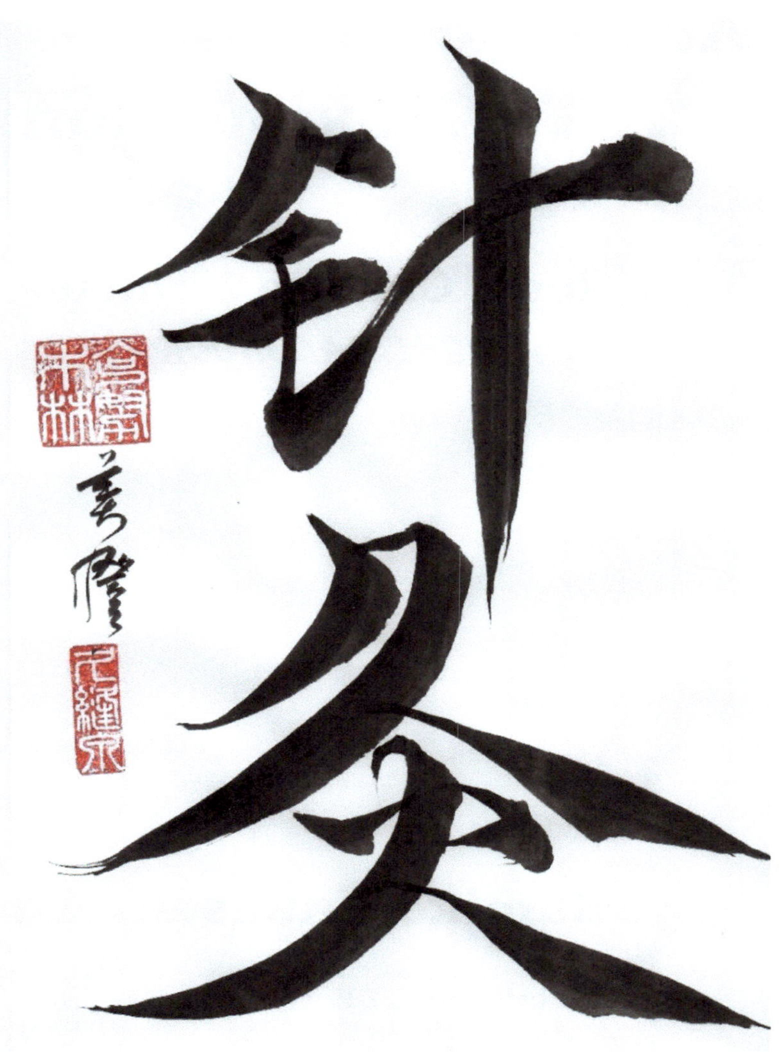

CONTENTS

INTRODUCTION

Traditional Chinese medicine has been used for over 3000 years in China, and it is still used to treat different kinds of disorders.

According to TCM, acupuncture is based on the balance between Yin and Yang in Chinese philosophy. "Life energy" that is "Qi" flows through channels in our body. Upon stimulation with specific places in the body with the single use of the needle gets the energy to flow, and it becomes better conditions.

Acupuncture is oriental medicine, which has no side effects. Acupuncture may prevent diseases by strengthening the immune system in the body. Acupuncture is done by inserting thin disposable needles into specific points relating to the internal organs. In this way the body is activated with flow of Qi (energy).

In Therapeutics of acupuncture, acupuncture points are the places where acupuncture needle is applied for the treatment of diseases. This acupuncture point location and the therapeutic result are related.

In the treatment of disease by acupuncture and moxibustion, the equipment is simple, but it shows effective result.

Sumiko Knudsen 克努森澄子

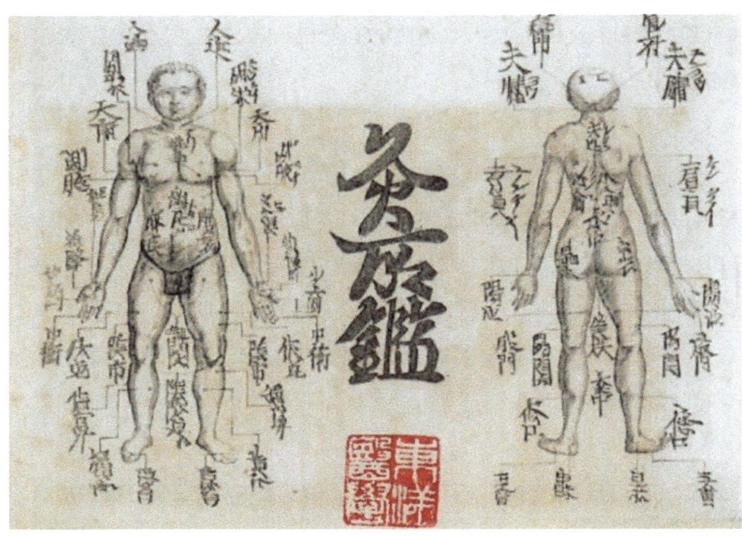

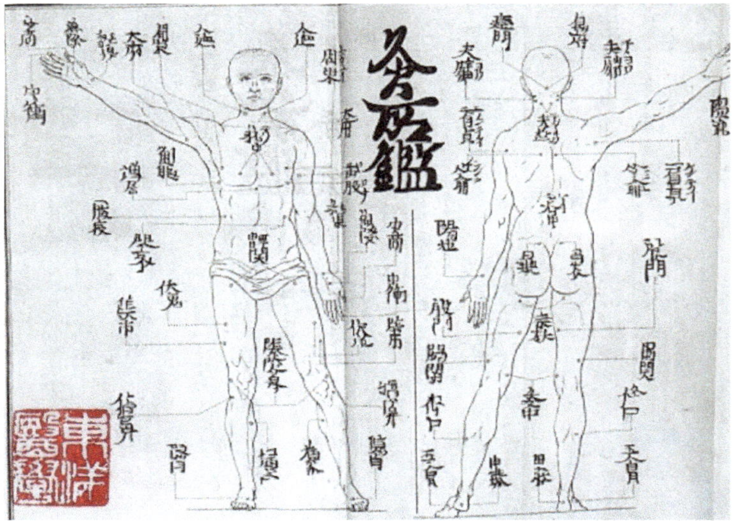

Points were used by Moxibustion about 1700.

CHARPTER 1 Acupuncture and Moxibustion

1. What is Acupuncture and Moxibustion?

Acupuncture and Moxibustion are two different of methods therapy. Acupuncture treatment is by puncturing certain points with metal needles on skin surface, and Moxibustion treatment is the application of heat produced by moxa-wool made from dry herbs over the points on the skin surface.
Even though materials for treatment are used in the two methods of different ways, therapeutic and preventive results are similarly achieved.

By those methods, Qi and Blood will be stimulated in the channels, and it achieves prevention and treatment of diseases.

Acupuncture and Moxibustion are often used at the same time for effectiveness for treatment in clinic, therefore it is called Acupuncture and Moxibustion.

2. Introduction of Acupuncture Points

Acupuncture points are the places where acupuncture needle is applied for the treatment of diseases.
Acupuncture points are related to Qi of the Zang-fu organs and meridians is transported to the body surface.

Acupuncture point is writtenas in Chinese word "Shuxue, 腧穴", and these Chinese characters mean respectively transport and hole.

Acupuncture points are not only the pathways for the circulation of Qi and Blood, but also response to diseases.

The locations of Acupuncture points are certainly related to physiological functions. Stimulating Acupuncture points in meridians of the affected area may be effective for each disease to approach the affected area.

To strengthen body resistance to prevent and treat diseases, proper techniques in Acupuncture and Moxibustion treatment are required.

3. Moxibustion

Moxibustion treats and prevents diseases by applying heat to points or certain locations of the human body. The material used is mainly moxa-wool in the form of a long stick or a small cone.

Moxa-wool is made of dry mugwort leaves. Moxa has the properties of warming, removing obstruction in the meridians, and eliminating Cold and Damp, thus promoting to the normal function of the organs.

There are three methods of application which are used with Moxa Cones, Moxa Sticks, and warming needles, respectively.

1. With Moxa Cone

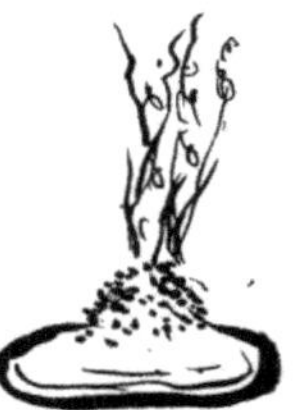

(1) Direct Moxibustion

Moxa cone is placed directly on the point. This method may lead to a local burn, blister, festering etc. If the patient feels a burning discomfort, remove the cone and place another one.

(2) Indirect Moxibustion
• Moxibustion with Ginger

Cut a slice of ginger about 0.5 cm thick and make some holes in it. Moxa cone is placed on top of this Ginger and the moxa cone is ignited.

This method relieves pain caused by Stomach and Spleen weakness such as abdominal pain, diarrhea, joint pain due to Yang deficiency.

• Moxibustion with Garlic

Cut a slice of garlic about 0.5 cm thick and make some holes in it. Moxa cone is placed on top of this garlic and the moxa cone is ignited.
This method is effective against tuberculosis, scrofula, ulcer with boils, insect bite etc.

• Moxibustion with Salt

This method is normally applied at the umbilicus REN-8 (Shenque 神阙). Apply salt to the level of the skin at the umbilicus, and place moxa cone on top of the salt, and then ignite it.
This method treats for abdominal pain, vomiting and diarrhea. This is to restore Yang from collapse.

2. With Moxa Sticks

(1) Mild-Warm Moxibustion

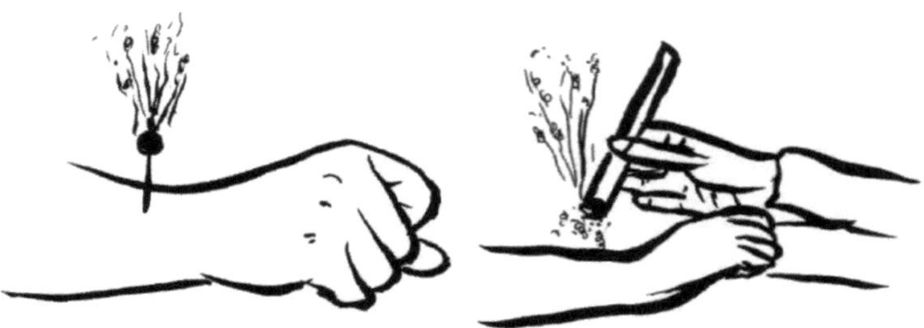

Apply an ignited moxa stick over the point of skin for about fifteen minutes until the local area become light red colour.

(2) Moxibustion on the needle area

Moxibustion is applied on the point where the needle stands. This functions to warm the meridians and promote the free flow of Qi and Blood.

(3) Moxibustion with warming needle

This is the method of acupuncture combined with moxibustion. This method functions to warm the meridians and promote the free flow of Qi and Blood to treat joints, numbness caused by Cold-Damp.

CHARPTER 2 Channels, Collaterals and Points

1. Methods of Acupuncture points location 腧穴定位的方法

There are three methods of Acupuncture point location which are used in clinic at present.

1-1. Anatomical Landmarks 骨度 折量定位法

Anatomical landmarks include 2 landmarks which are Fixed landmarks and Moving landmarks.

1) Fixed landmarks

Fixed landmarks which would not change with body movement. It is five sensory organs, hair, nails, nipple, umbilicus, and prominence and depression of the bones. They are for example, Ex-1 印堂 (Yintang), DU-25 素髎 (Suliao) and Ren-8 神阙 (Shenque).

2) Moving landmarks

It refers to appear when the part of body keeps in a specific position, and for example, when the arm is flexed and the cubital crease appear, LI-11 曲池 (Quchi). SI-3 后溪 (Houxi) which is made from fist, the point is at the end of the distal transverse crease of the palm.

2. Proportional Measurements 指寸定位法

Human body which is width and length of various portions of the body are divided respectively into definite numbers of proportional measurement. These are standard on any sexes, age, and body sizes for patients.

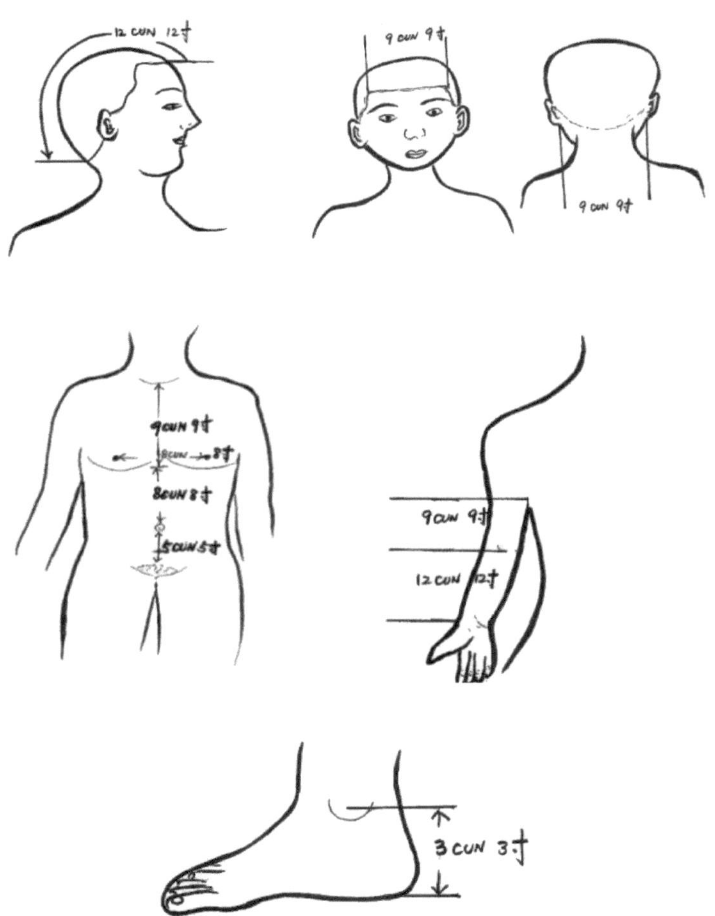

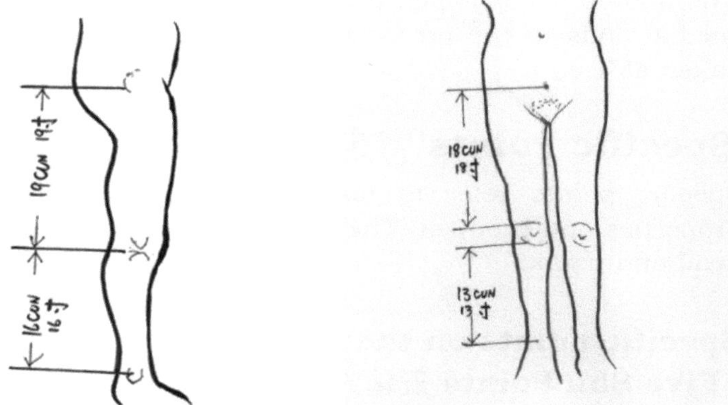

3. Finger Measurements 指寸定位法

1) Thumb measurement

The width of the thumb is taken as one cun.

2) Four finger measurement

The width of the four fingers such as index, middle, ring and little are used. Those fingers should be close together to the middle finger and are taken as three cun.

3) Middle finger measurement

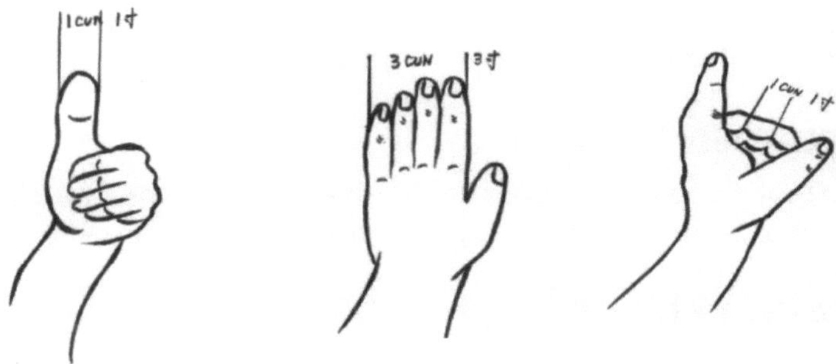

The middle finger is flexed, and the distance between two medial ends of the crease of the interphalangeal joint is taken as 1 cun.

2. Specific Points 特定穴

Specific points refer to fourteen channels which have properties and grouped. They are classified into limbs and head and trunk.

1. Specific points on the Limbs
1.1 Five Shu Points 五输穴

each of the twelve main channels has five Shu   points which are Jing-Well, Ying-Spring, Shu-Stream, Jing-River and He-Sea. In addition, there are Lower He-Sea points.

1.2 Yuan-Primary Points 原穴

Each of the twelve main channels has a Yuan-Primary point, and they are taken to treat disorders of the Zang-Fu organs.

1.3 Luo-Connecting Points 络穴

Each of the twelve main channels has a Luo-connecting point, and they are taken to treat disorders of the two exterior-interior related channels.

1.4 Xi-Cleft Points 郄穴

Xi-Cleft points where the Qi and Blood of the channel are deeply converged are used to treat acute disorders.

1.5 Ashi Points 啊是穴

Ashi points are the points of pain. "Where there is a painful spot, there is an acupuncture point" by Yellow emperor.

1.6 He-Sea Points 合穴

These points are all located below the knees and elbows and are used to treat disorders involving the face, head and trunk.

1.7 The Lower He-Sea Points 下合穴

These points are for the treatment of the disorders of the six fu organs.

1.8 Eight Confluent Points 八会穴

These points are located on the trunk and four limbs below the knees and elbow. They are P-6 (Neiguan 内关), SP-4 (Gongsun 公孙), SI-3 (Houxi 后溪), BL-62 (Shenmai 申脉), SJ-5 (Waiguan 外关), GB-41 (Zulinqi 足临泣), LU-7 (Lieque 列缺), KI-6 (Zhaohai 照海).

2. Specific points on the Head and Trunk
2.1 Back-Shu Points 背俞穴

Back-Shu points are specific points on the back where the Qi of the Zang-Fu organs is infused.

2.2 Front-Mu Points 募穴

Front-Mu points are on the chest and abdomen where the Qi of the Zang-Fu organs is infused.

2.3 Crossing Points 交会穴

Most of them are located on the head, face and trunk, except a few which are located on the lower limbs. These points are used to treat diseases related to the meridian proper.

3. The 14 Channels and their Points 十四经穴的定位

I. The Lung Channel of Hand Taiyin
手太阴肺经经穴

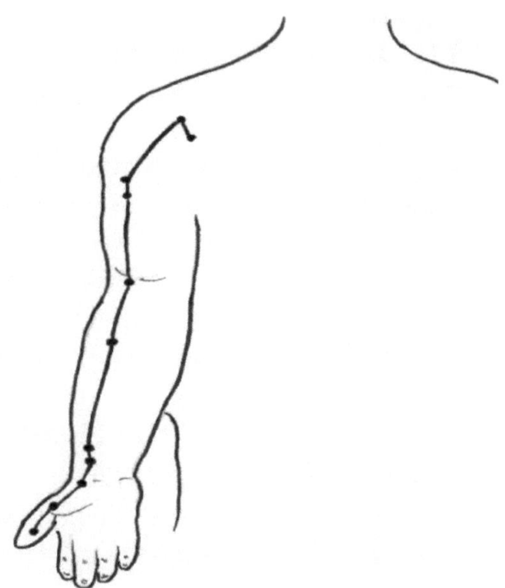

Starts on the chest near the armpit and it goes continuously downward the forearm to end of medial side of the tip of the thumb. It contains 11 different acupoints.

LU-1 (Zhongfu 中府)
* **Front-Mu point**

Indications

Cough, Asthma, chest pain, fullness of the chest.

Location

On the lateral aspect of the chest in the first intercostal space, 1 cun directly below LU-2, 6 cun lateral to the anterior midline.

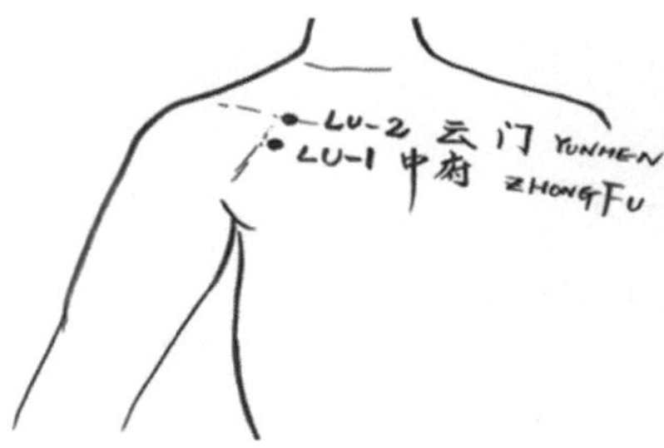

LU-2 (Yunmen 云门)

Indications

Cough, Asthma, pain in the chest, fullness of the chest, shoulder, and arm pain.

Location

On the antero-lateral aspect of the chest, there is a depression the shape of triangle at the lower lateral of the clavicle, 6 cun lateral to the midline.

LU-3 (Tianfu 天府)

Indications

Asthma, Epistaxis, medial aspect of the upper arm pain.

Location

On the medial aspect of the upper arm, 3 cun inferior to the end of the axillary fold, radial side of the biceps brachii.

When raising the arm forward, touch the radial side of the biceps brachii with the tip of the nose.

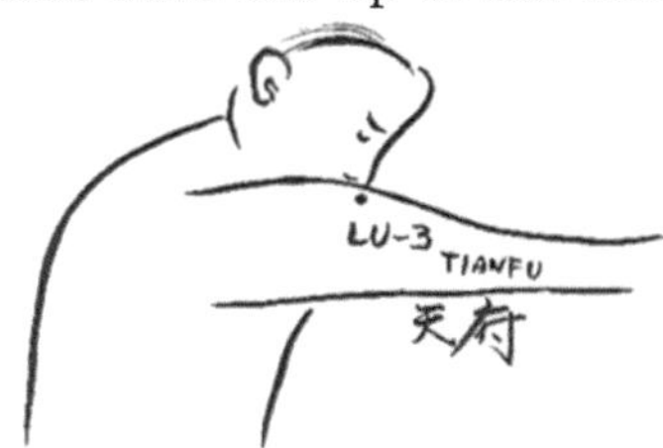

LU-4 (Xiabai 侠白)

Indications

Cough, fullness in the Chest, medial aspect of the upper arm pain.

Location

With the upper arm flexed, it is located 1 cun below LU-3.

LU-5 (Chize 尺泽)

- **He Sea point**

Indications

Cough, Asthma, Dyspnea, Hemoptysis, fullness of the chest, afternoon fever, sore throat, spasmodic pain of the elbow and arm.

Location

On the transverse cubital crease, in the depression at the radial side of the tendon of biceps brachii.

LU-6 (Kongzui 孔最)

- **Xi-Cleft point**

Indications

Hemoptysis, cough, dyspnea, sore throat, hemorrhoids, aphonia, pain of the arm and elbow, headache.

Location

On the medial border of the radius, along the line connection LU-5, 5 cun below. 7 cun above the LU-9.

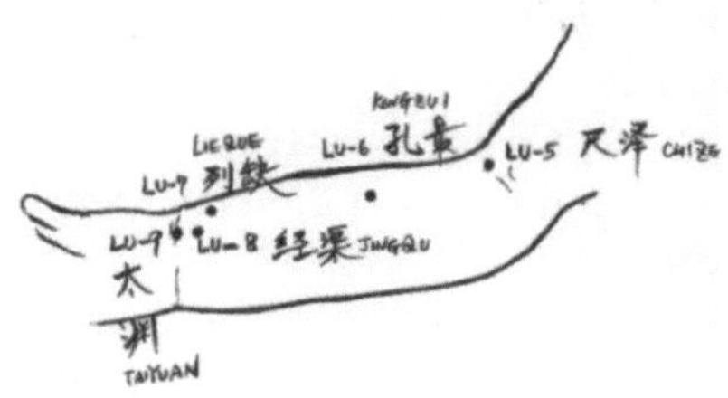

LU-7 (Lieque 列缺)

- **Luo-Connecting point**

Indications

Cough, asthma, migraine, hemoptysis, sore throat, stiff neck, toothache, feverish urination, pain in the penis and feverish sensation in the palms.

Location

On the radial aspect of the forearm 1.5 cun above the transverse crease of the wrist between two tendons.

When the index fingers and thumbs of both hands are crossed with the other hand, LU-7 is right under the tip of the index finger.

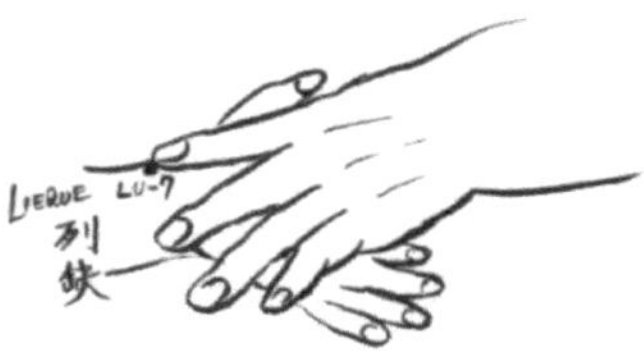

LU-8 (Jingqu 经渠)

Indications

Cough, asthma, sore throat, pain in the chest, pain in the wrist.

Location

1 cun above the transverse crease of the wrist, in the depression on the lateral side of the radial artery.

LU-9 (Taiyuan 太渊)

- **Yuan-Primary point**

Indications

Cough, asthma, sore throat, palpitation, pain in the chest, wrist, arm.

Location

At the radial end of transvers crease of the wrist, in the depression on the radial side of the radial artery.

LU-10 (Yuji 鱼际)

Indications

Cough, hemoptysis, sore throat, aphonia, loss of voice, feverish sensation in the palms.

Location

At the radial aspect of the midpoint of the first metacarpal bone, on the junction of the red and white skin.

LU-11 (Shaoshang 少商)

- **Jing-Well point**

Indications

Cough, asthma, sore throat, epistaxis, abdominal fullness, mania, pain of the thumb.

Location

On the radial side of the thumb, 0.1 cun from the corner of the nail.

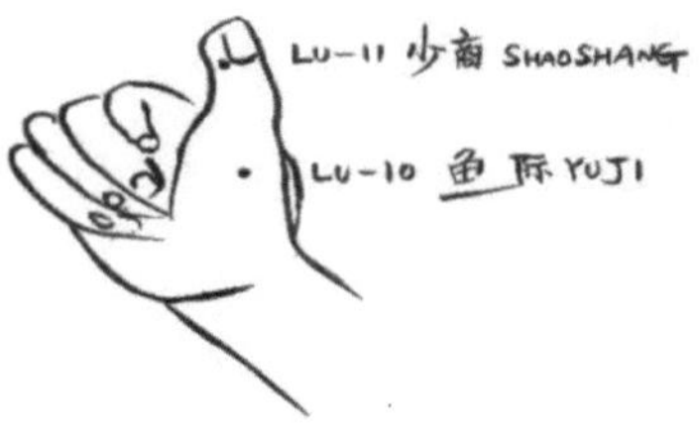

II. The Large Intestine Channel of Hand-Yangming 手阳明大肠经经穴

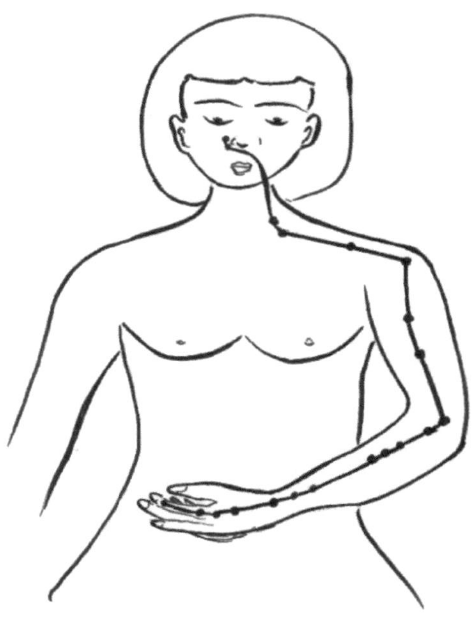

Starts at the tip of the index finger along the upper side of the arm to the highest point of the shoulder, runs upward to the neck, passes through the cheek to the nose. It contains 20 different acupoints.

LI-1 (Shangyang 商阳)
- **Jing-Well point**

Indications

> Apoplexy, coma, toothache, deafness, numbness of fingers, high fever.

Location

On the radial side of the index finger, 0.1 cun beside the corner of the nail.

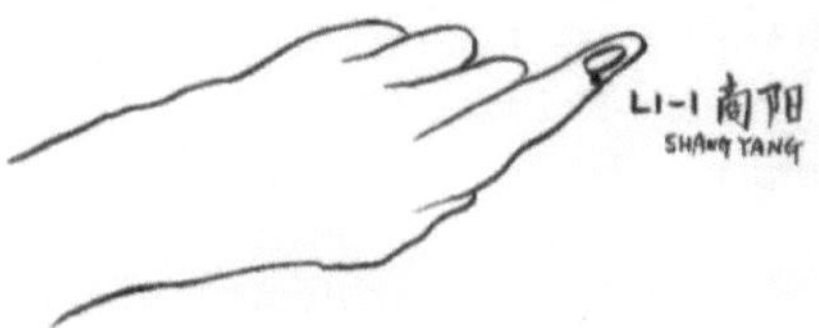

LI-2 (Erjian 二间)

Indications

Toothache, sore throat, blurring of vision, facial paralysis, numbness of fingers.

Location

On the radial side of the index finger, in the depression distal to the second metacarpal-phalangeal joint. Point locates slightly flexed.

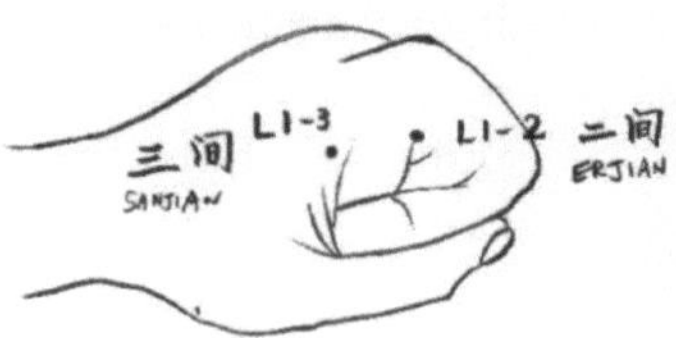

LI-3 (Sanjian 三间)

Indications

Toothache, sore throat, epistaxis, swelling and pain of the dorsum of hand, numbness of fingers.

Location

On the radial side of the index finger, in the depression proximal to the second metacarpal-phalangeal joint.

LI-4 (Hegu 合谷)

- **Yuan-Primary point**

Indication

Swelling, redness and pain of eyes, headache, facial paralysis, epistaxis, sore throat, deafness, toothache, swelling of the face, common cold, cough, paralysis and spasm of fingers, infantile convulsion, irregular menstruation, delayed labour, obstruction syndrome in apoplexy, weakness and motor impairment.

Location

On the dorsum of the hand between the first and second metacarpal bones, locate the point to stretch both thumbs and index finger of the left hand, place the transvers crease of the interphalangeal joint of the right thumb on the margin of the web between the left hand. The point is where the tip of the thumb touches.

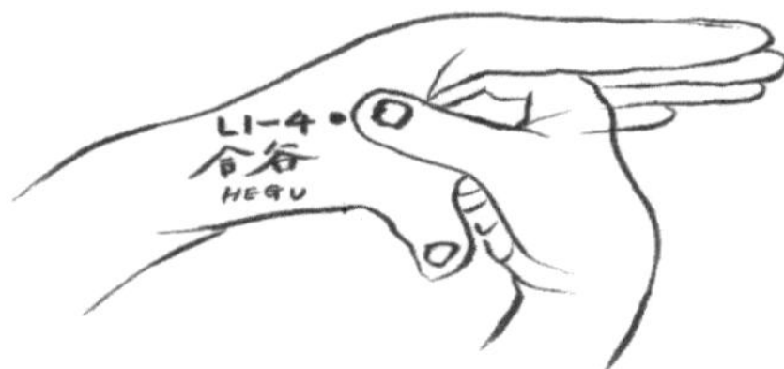

LI-5 (Yangxi 阳溪)
Indications

Headache, tinnitus, deafness, mania, epilepsy, spasmodic pain in the wrist, toothache, redness, pain, and swelling in the eyes.

Location

On the radial side of the wrist, when the thumb is tilted upward, it is the depression between the tendons of extensor pollicis longus and brevis.

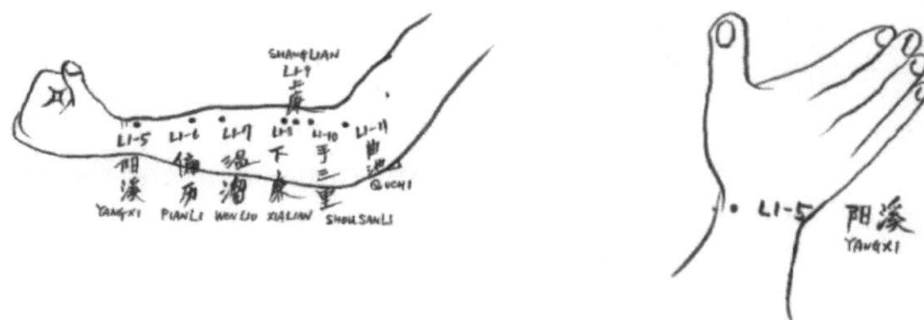

LI-6 (Pianli 偏历)

- **Luo-Connecting point**

Indications

Tinnitus, deafness, redness of the eye, spasmodic pain in the arm and hand, epistaxis, facial paralysis, sore throat, edema.

Location

On the radial side of dorsal surface of the forearm, 3 cun proximal to the wrist crease.

LI-7 (Wenliu 温溜)

- **Xi-Cleft point**

Indications

Headache, epistaxis, sore throat, abdominal pain, pain in the shoulder and arm.

Location

On the radial side of dorsal surface of the forearm, 5 cun proximal to the wrist crease.

LI-8 (Xialian 下廉)

Indications

Abdominal pain, pain in the elbow and arm, motor impairment of the upper limbs.

Location

On the radial side of dorsal surface of the forearm, 4 cun distal to the cubital crease.

LI-9 (Shanglian 上廉)

Indications

Motor impairment of the upper limbs, numbness of the hand and arm, pain in shoulder and arm, abdominal pain.

Location

On the radial side of dorsal surface of the forearm, 3 cun distal to the cubital crease.

LI-10 (Shousanli 手三里)

Indications

Toothache, swelling of the cheek, abdominal pain, borborygmus, diarrhea, paralysis of the upper limbs, pain in the shoulder and back.

Location

On the radial side of dorsal surface of the forearm, 2 cun distal to the cubital crease.

LI-11 (Quchi 曲池)

- **He-Sea point**

Indications

Toothache, redness and pain of eyes, sore throat, abdominal pain, diarrhea, paralysis of the upper limbs, spasmodic pain of the elbow and arm, febrile diseases, hypertension, urticaria.

Location

In the depression at the lateral end of the transverse cubital crease.

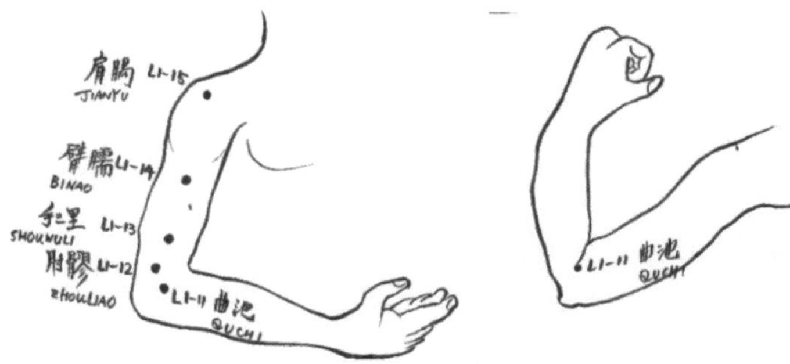

LI-12 (Zhouliao 肘髎)

Indications

Numbness, spasmodic pain in the elbow and arm.

Location

On the lateral side of the upperarm, 1 cun above to LI-11(Quchi 曲池).

LI-13 (Shouwuli 手五里)

Indications

Spasmodic pain in the elbow and arm, scrofula.

Location

On the lateral side of the upperarm, 3 cun above to LI-11(Quchi 曲池).

LI-14 (Binao 臂臑)

Indications

Pain in the shoulder and arm, stiff neck, shortsightedness, night blindness, scrofula.

Location

On the lateral side of the upperarm, on the line joining LI-11 (Quchi 曲池) and LI-15 (Jianyu 肩髃), 7 cun above LI-11 (Quchi 曲池).

LI-15 (Jianyu 肩髃)

Indications

Pain in the shoulder and arm, flaccidity of the upper limbs, urticaria, scrofula.

Location

On the shoulder, in the depression anterior border of the acromioclavicular point.

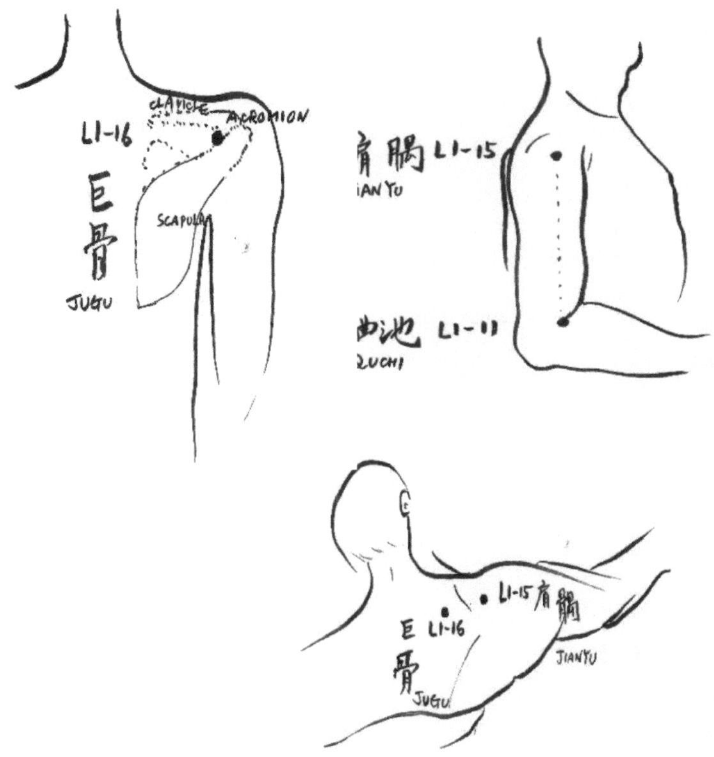

LI-16 (Jugu 巨骨)

Indications

Pain and motor impairment of the upper extremities, pain in the shoulder.

Location

On the shoulder, in the depression between the acromial extremity of the clavicle and the scapular spine.

LI-17 (Tianding 天鼎)

Indications

Sudden loss of the voice, sore throat, scrofula, goiter.

Location

On the lateral side of the neck, at the posterior border of the sternocleidomastoid muscle. 1 cun inferior to Li-18 (Futu 扶突).

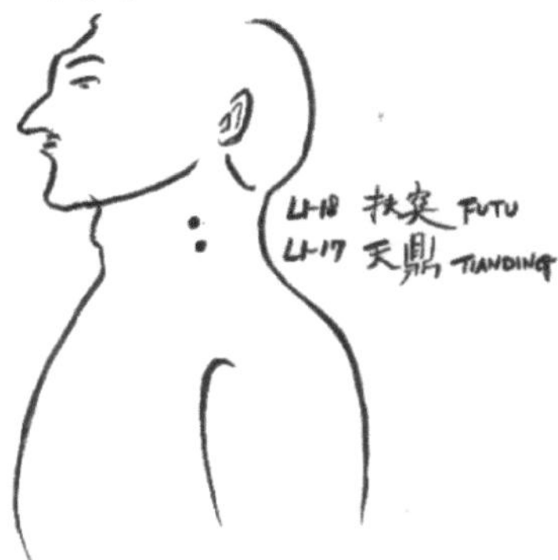

LI-18 (Futu 扶突)

Indications

Cough, asthma, sore throat, scrofula, goiter, sudden loss of the voice.

Location

On the lateral side of the neck, level with the tip of Adam's apple between the anterior and posterior borders of the sternocleidomastoid muscle.

LI-19 (Kouheliao 口禾髎)

Indications

Nose disorders, epistaxis, deviation of the mouth.

Location

Below the lateral border of the nostril and near the upper lip, at the level of Du-26 (Renzong 人中).

LI-20 (Yingxiang 迎香)

Indications

Nasal obstruction, epistaxis, deviation of the mouth, itching and swelling of the face.

Location

In the naso-labial groove, at the level of the midpoint of the ala nasi.

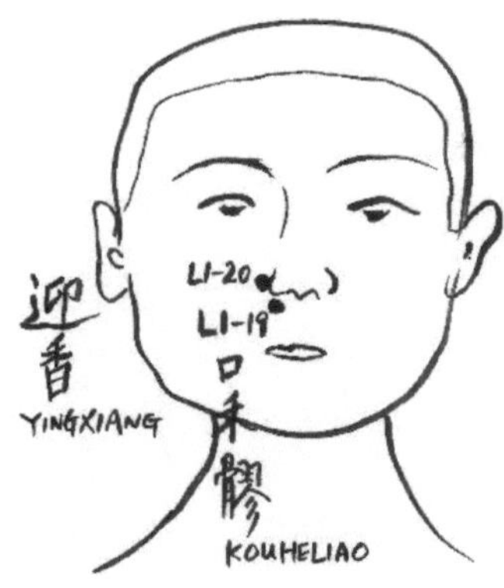

III. The Stomach Channel of Foot-Yangming 足阳明胃经经穴

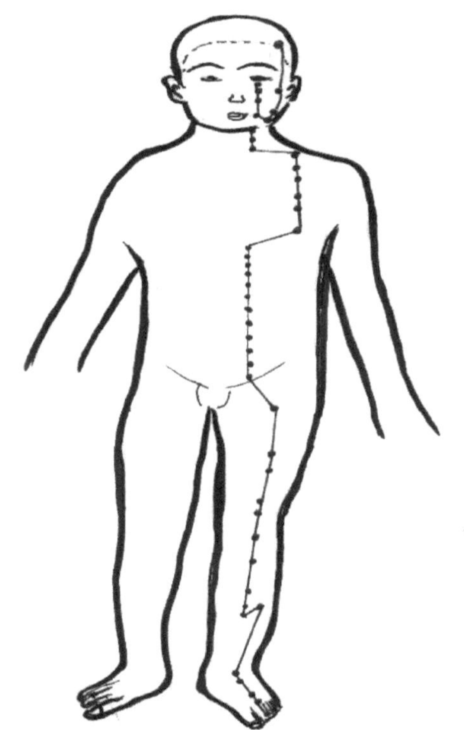

Starts below the pupil of the eye and then to the nose to the jaw, where it splits. The one goes up the scalp but the other one runs down to the neck, chest, abdomen, thigh and through down to the side of the tip of the second toe. It contains 45 different acupoints.

ST-1 (Chengqi 承泣)

Indications

Redness, pain and itching of the eye, twitching eyelids, facial paralysis.

Location

With the eyes looking straight forward, the point is directly   below the pupil between the eyeball and the infraorbital ridge.

ST-2 (Sibai 四白)

Indications

Redness, itching and pain of eyes, cataract, facial paralysis, headache, vertigo, twitching of eyelids.

Location

With the eyes looking straight forward, the point is directly below the pupil, in the depression of the infraorbital foramen.

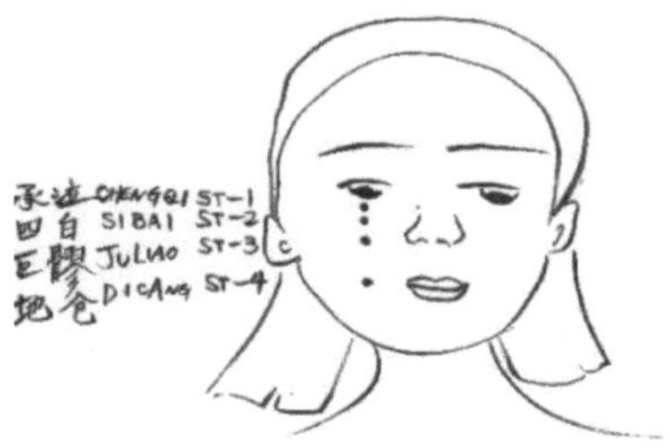

ST-3 (Juliao 巨髎)

Indications

Facial paralysis, twitching of eyelids, epitaxis, toothache, swelling of lips and cheeks.

Location

With the eyes looking straight forward, the point is directly below the pupil, level of the lower border of the ala nasi on the lateral side of the naso-labial groove.

ST-4 (Dicang 地仓)

Indications

Twitching of eyelids, deviation of the mouth, toothache.

Location

Lateral corner of the mouth.

ST-5 (Daying 大迎)

Indications

Facial paralysis, swelling of the cheek, pain in the face, toothache.

Location

Anterior to the angle of the mandible, in the depression at the anterior border of the masseter muscle.

ST-6 (Jiache 颊车)

Indications

Lockjaw, swelling of the cheeks, toothache, swelling of the cheek and face.

Location

One finger-breadth anterior and superior to the angle of the mandible.

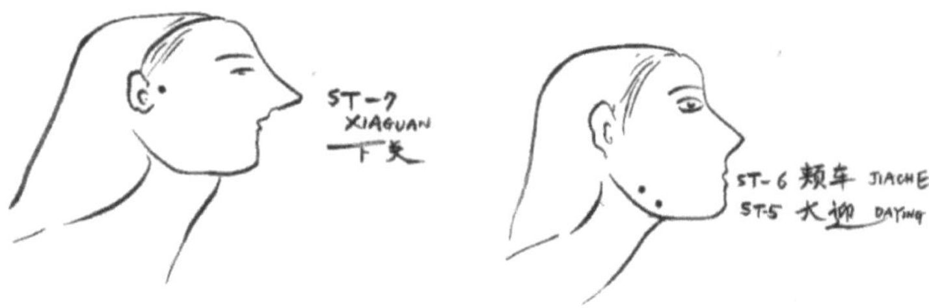

ST-7 (Xiaguan 下关)

Indications

Deafness, Tinnitus, lockjaw, toothache, motor impairment of the jaw, pain in the face, facial paralysis.

Location

Anterior to the ear on the face, in the depression between zygomatic arch and mandibular notch.

ST-8 (Touwei 头维)

Indications

Headache, vertigo, blurring of vision, lacrimation.

Location

0.5 cun above the anterior hairline at the corner of the forehead.

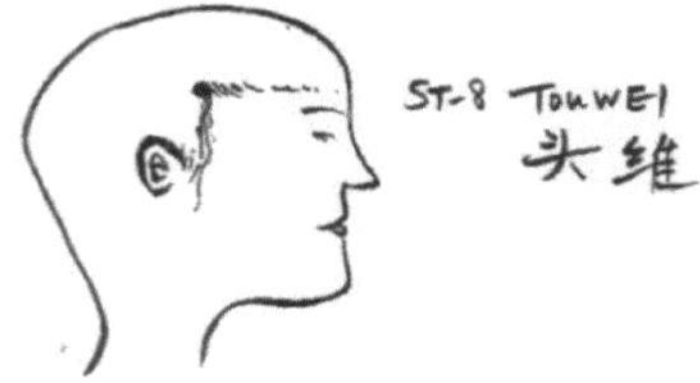

ST-9 (Renying 人迎)

Indications

Sore throat, asthma, scrofula, goiter, hypertension, dizziness.

Location

Level with the tip of Adam apple, on the anterior border of the sternocleidomastoid muscle where the common carotid artery is palpable.

ST-10 (Shuitu 水突)

Indications

Sore throat, asthma, cough.

Location

On the neck, on the anterior border of the sternocleidomastoid muscle, midpoint of the line ST-9 (Renying 人迎) and ST-11 (Qishe 气舍).

ST-11 (Qishe 气舍)

Indications

Sore throat, asthma, hiccup, goiter.

Location

On the neck, superior to the medial end of the clavicle, directly under ST-9 (Renying 人迎) between the sternal and clavicular heads of the sternocleidomastoid muscle.

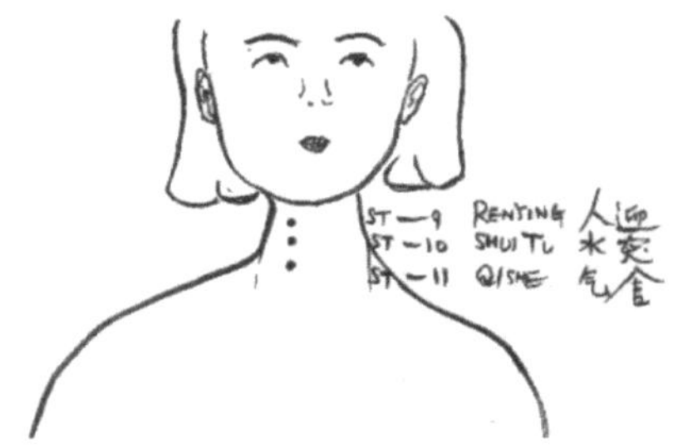

ST-12 (Quepen 缺盆)

Indications

Cough, asthma, sore throat, pain in the supraclavicular fossa.

Location

This point is at the midpoint of the supraclavicular fossa, 4 cun lateral to the midline.

ST-13 (Qihu 气户)

Indications

Asthma, cough, fullness in the chest, hiccup, pain in the chest, hypochondorium.

Location

This point is at the midpoint of the lower border of the clavicle, directly below ST-12 (Quepen 缺盆). 4 cun lateral to the midline.

ST-14 (Kufang 库房)

Indications

Cough, Sensation of fullness and pain in the chest.

Location

On the chest, in the first intercostal space, 4 cun lateral to the anterior midline.

ST-15 (Wuyi 屋翳)

Indications

Cough, asthma, fullness and pain in the chest and costal region, mastitis.

Location

On the chest, in the second intercostal space, 4 cun lateral to the anterior midline.

ST-16 (Yingchuang 膺窗)

Indications

Cough, asthma, fullness and pain in the chest and hypochondrium, mastitis.

Location

On the chest, in the third intercostal space, 4 cun lateral to the anterior midline.

ST-17 (Ruxhong 乳中)

Location

On the chest, in the fourth intercostal space, at the corner of the nipple, 4 cun lateral to the anterior midline.

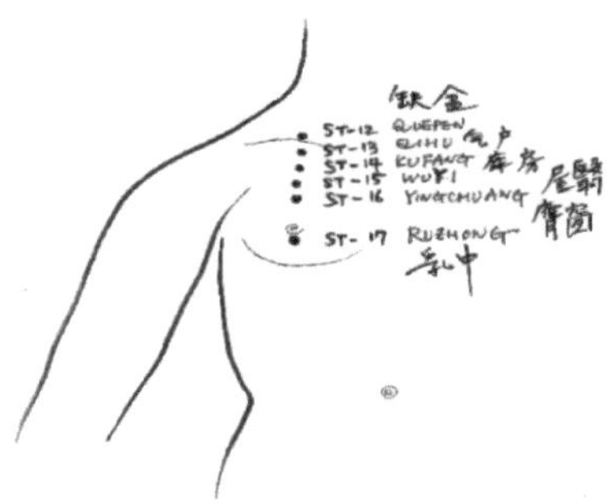

ST-18 (Rugen 乳根)

Indications

Cough, asthma, hiccup, chest pain breast abscess.

Location

On the chest, directly below the nipple, in the fifth intercostal space.

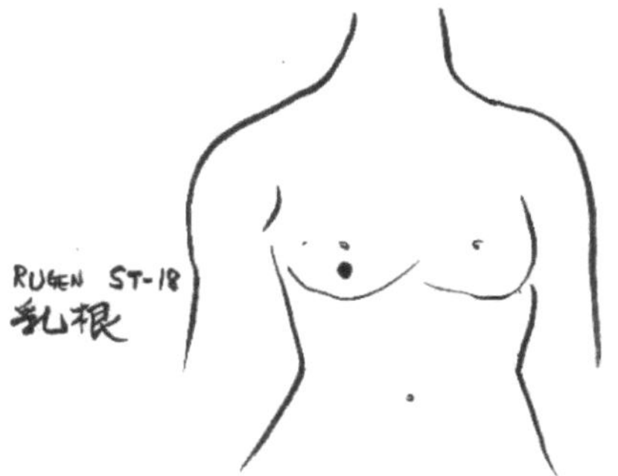

ST-19 (Burong 不容)

Indications

Abdominal distension, gastric pain, vomiting, anorexia.

Location

On the upper abdomen, 6 cun above the umbilicus, 2 cun lateral to the anterior midline.

ST-20 (Chengman 承满)

Indications

Abdominal distension, gastric pain, vomiting, anorexia.

Location

On the upper abdomen, 5 cun above the umbilicus, 2 cun lateral to the anterior midline.

ST-21 (Liangmen 梁门)

Indications

Abdominal distension, diarrhea, vomiting, stomachache, anorexia.

Location

On the abdomen, 4 cun above the umbilicus, 2 cun lateral to the anterior midline.

ST-22 (Guanmen 关门)

Indications

Pain and abdominal distension, diarrhea, borborygmus, anorexia, edema.

Location

On the abdomen, 3 cun above the umbilicus, 2 cun lateral to the anterior midline.

ST-23 (Taiyi 太乙)

Indications

Gastric pain, Irritability, Mania.

Location

On the abdomen, 2 cun above the umbilicus, 2 cun lateral to the anterior midline.

ST-24 (Huaroumen 滑肉门)

Indications

Gastric pain, vomiting, mania.

Location

On the abdomen, 1 cun above the umbilicus, 2 cun lateral to the anterior midline.

ST-25 (Tianshu 天枢)

- **Front-Mu point of the Large Intestine.**

Indications

Abdominal distension, borborygmus, diarrhea, pain around the umbilicus, dysentery, irregular menstruation, edema.

Location

On the addomen, 2 cun lateral to the umbilicus.

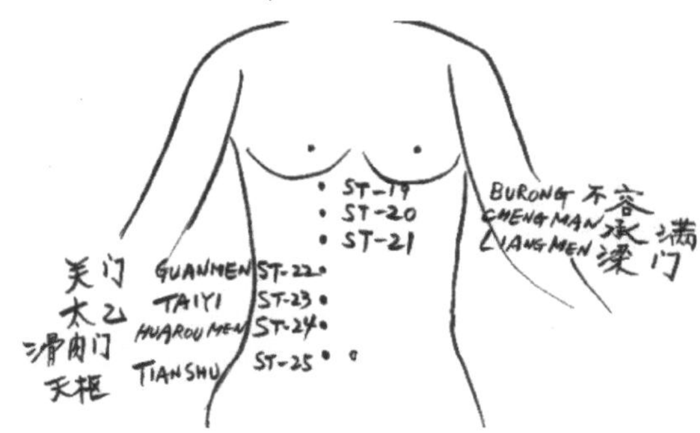

ST-26 (Wailing 外陵)

Indications

Abdominal pain, hernia, dysmenorrhea.

Location

On the lower abdomen, 1 cun below the umbilicus, 2 cun lateral to the anterior midline.

ST-27 (Daju 大巨)

Indications

Helnia, Lower abdominal distension, dysuria, seminal emission.

Location

On the lower abdomen, 2 cun below the umbilicus, 2 cun lateral to the anterior midline.

ST-28 (Shuidao 水道)

Indications

Abdominal distension, hernia, dysuria, dysmenorrhea, edema.

Location

On the lower abdomen, 3 cun below the umbilicus, 2 cun lateral to the anterior midline.

ST-29 (Guilai 归来)

Indications

Irregular menstruation, leukorrhea, hernia, abdominal pain, prolapse of uterus.

Location

On the lower abdomen, 4 cun below the umbilicus, 2 cun lateral to the anterior midline.

ST-30 (Qichong 气冲)

Indications

Abdominal pain, irregular menstruation, hernia, impotence, swelling and pain of the external genitalia.

Location

On the lower abdomen, 5 cun below the umbilicus, 2 cun lateral to the anterior midline.

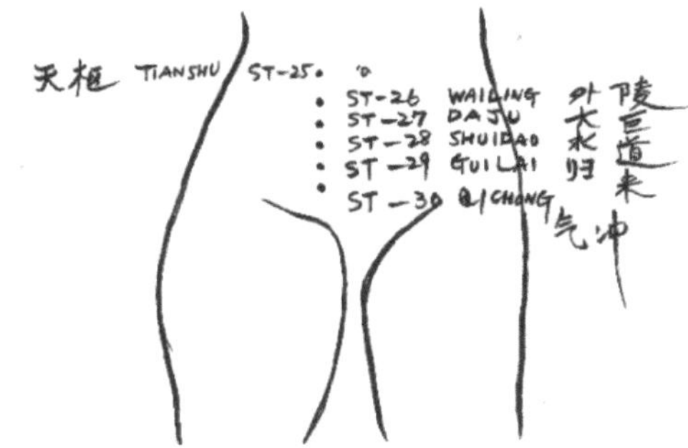

ST-31 (Biguan 髀关)

Indications

Pain in the thigh, motor impairment, numbness, pain of the lower extremities, muscular atrophy.

Location

On the upper thigh, on the line connecting the anterosuperior iliac spine and the superiolateral border of the patella.

Sitting upright with the knee flexed, two-finger width down directly from the inguinal groove, directing the midline of the patella.

ST-32 (Futu 伏兔)

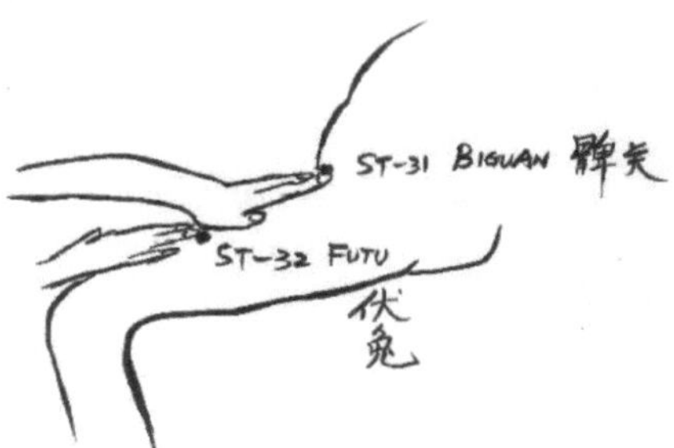

Indications

Pain in the lumbar and iliac region, paralysis of the lower limbs, hernia, beriberi.

Location

On the thigh, on the line connecting anterior superior iliac spine and the lateral border of the patella, 6 cun above the laterosuperior border of the patella.

Sitting upright with the knee flexed, puts the center of the transverse crease of the wrist on the center of the upper border of the patella with closed fingers on the thigh. The point is where the tip of the middle finger.

ST-33 (Yinshi 阴市)

Indications

Numbness, soreness, motor impairment of the leg and knee.

Location

On the thigh, the point is 3 cun above the laterosuperior border of patella. On the line connecting the anterior superior lilac spine and the lateral superior border of the patella.

ST-34 (Liang 梁丘)

- **Xi-Cleft point of the Stomach channel.**

Indications

Stomachache, swelling and pain of the knee and paralysis of the lower limbs, breast abscess, hematuria.

Location

On the thigh, 2 cun above the superiolateral border of the patella.

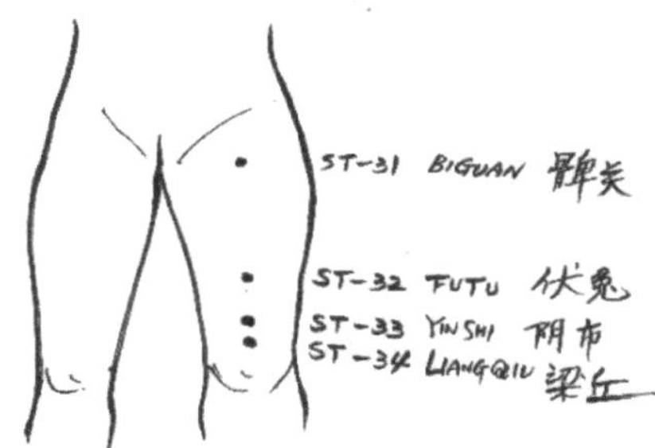

ST-35 (Dubi 犊鼻)

Indication

Pain of knee, paralysis of the lower limbs, beriberi.

Location

On the knee, in the depression lateral to the patella and the patellar ligament.

ST-36 (Zusanli 足三里)

- **He-Sea point of the Stomach channel.**

Indicatons

Abdominal distension, vomiting, stomachache, diarrhea, constipation, edema, dysentery, paralysis of lower limbs, beriberi, emaciation, cough, asthma, mania, insomnia.

Location

3 cun inferior to ST-35 (Dubi 犊鼻), one finger breadth (middle finger) lateral to the anterior crest of the tibia.

ST-37 (Shangjuxu 上巨虚)

- **Lower He-Sea point of the Large Intestine.**

Indications

Borborygmus, abdominal pain, diarrhea, constipation, intestinal abscess, beriberi, flaccidity, paralysis.

Location

On the lower leg, 6 cun inferior to ST-35 (Dubi 犊鼻), one finger- breadth (middle finger) lateral to the anterior crest of the tibia.

ST-38 (Tiaokou 条口)

Indications

Pain in the shoulder and arm, epigastric pain, numbness of the knee and leg, motor impairment of the foot and shoulder.

Location

On the lower leg, 8 cun inferior to ST-35 (Dubi 犊鼻), one finger breadth (middle finger) lateral to the anterior crest of the tibia.

ST-39 (Xiajuxu 下巨虚)

- **Lower He-Sea point of the Small Intestine.**
- **Point of the Sea of Blood.**

Indications

Lower abdominal pain, diarrhea, numbness and paralysis of the lower extremities, breast abscess.

Location

On the lower leg, 9 cun inferior to ST-35 (Dubi 犊鼻), one finger- breadth (middle finger) lateral to the anterior crest of the tibia.

ST-40 (Fenglong 丰隆)

- **Luo-Connecting point of the Stomach channel.**

Indications

Vomiting, Edema, constipation, headache, vertigo, dizziness, cough, asthma, epilepsy, paralysis of the lower extremities, muscular atrophy.

Location

On the lower leg, 8 cun superior to the prominence of the lateral malleolus, lateral to ST-38 (Tiaokou 条口), two finger breadths lateral to the anterior crest of the tibia.

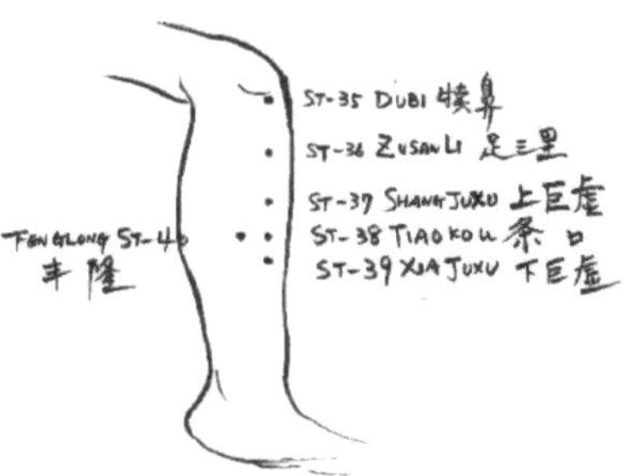

ST-41 (Jiexi 解溪)

Indications

Headache, vertigo, depressive and manic psychosis, constipation, abdominal distension, swelling and pain of ankle joint, syndromes of lower limbs.

Location

Midpoint of the dorsum of the foot at the transverse malleolus, in a depression between the tendons of extensor hallucis longus and extensor digitorum longus.

ST-41 (Jiexi 解溪)

Indications

Headache, vertigo, constipation, abdominal distension, epilepsy, swelling and pain of ankle joint, paralysis of the lower extremities, muscular atrophy, depressive and manic psychosis.

Location

Midpoint of the dorsum of the foot at the transverse malleolus, in a depression between the tendons of extensor hallucis longus and extensor digitorum longus.

ST-42 (Chongyang 冲阳)

- **Yuan-Source point of the Stomach channel.**

Indications

Swelling of cheeks, toothache, depressive and manic psychosis, epilepsy, impairment of the foot, epilepsy, muscular atrophy, epilepsy, flaccidity of foot.

Location

Highest point on the dorsum of the foot, in the depression distal to the junction of the second and third metatarsal bones.

ST-43 (Xiangu 陷谷)

Indications

Abdominal pain, swelling of cheeks, pain of the eyes, febrile disease, swelling and pain of the dorsum of foot.

Location

On the dorsum of the foot, between the second and third metatarsal bones, 1 cun proximal to ST-44 (Neiting 内庭).

ST-44 (Neiting 内庭)

Indications

Toothache, pain in the face, sore throat, stomachache, epistaxis, abdominal distension, constipation, dysentery, diarrhea, swelling and pain of dorsum of foot, febrile disease.

Location

On the dorsum of the foot, between the second and third toes, at the end of the vertical skin crease of the web.

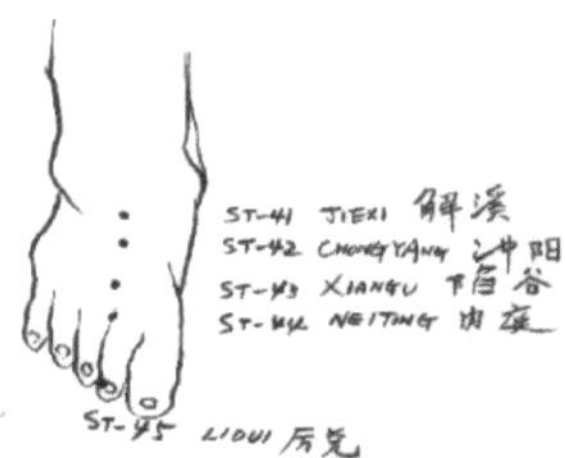

ST-45 (Lidui 厉兑)

- **Jing-Well point.**

Indications

Toothache, facial swelling, sore throat, epistaxis, Mania, febrile disease.

Location

On the lateral side of the 2nd toe, 0.1 cun beside the corner of the nail.

IV. The Spleen Channel of Foot-Taiyin
足太阴脾经经穴

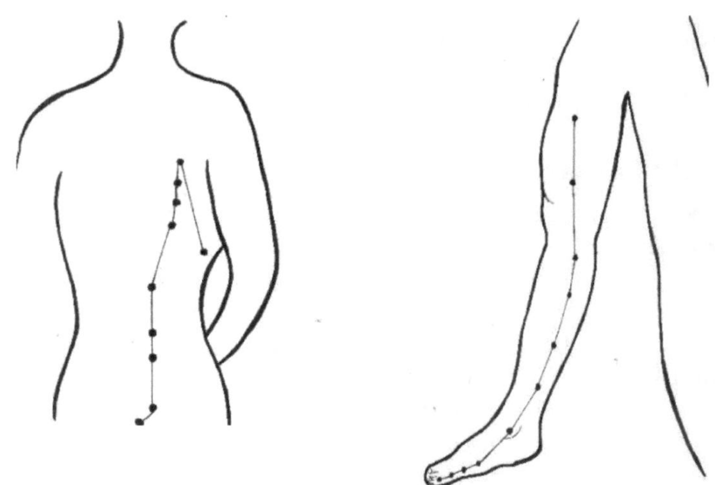

Starts from the tip of the big toe, passing through the anterior medial aspect of the knee and thigh, and enters the abdomen, then up the ribs to a point on the chest below the armpit. It contains 21 different acupoints.

SP-1 (Yinbai 隐白)

- **Jing-Well point.**

Indications

Abdominal distension, apoplexy, convulsion, mental disorders, metrorrhagia, uterine bleeding, bloody stools.

Location

On the medial side of the big toe, 0.1 cun beside the corner of the nail.

58

SP-2 (Dadu 大都)

Indications

Abdominal pain and distension, vomiting, diarrhea, febrile disease, constipation, dysphoria.

Location

On the medial side of the big toe, in the depression distal and inferior to the first metatarso-phalangeal joint.

SP-3 (Taibai 太白)

- **Yuan -Source point of the Spleen channel.**

Indications

Abdominal distension, stomachache, vomiting, diarrhea, constipation, edema, pain of joints, beriberi, heaviness of the body.

Location

On the medial side of the foot, in the depression proximal and inferior to the first metatarso-phalangeal joint.

SP-4 (Gongsun 公孙)

- **Luo-Connecting point of the Spleen channel.**

Indications

Abdominal distension, diarrhea, edema, vomiting, dysentery, stomachache, insomnia, dysphoria, borborygmus.

Location

On the medial side of the foot, in the depression distal and inferior to the base of the first metatarsal bone.

SP-5 (Shangqiu 商丘)

Indications

Abdominal distension, constipation, diarrhea, borborygmus, stiffness and pain of the tongue, hemorrhoid, pain in the foot and ankle.

Location

On the medial side of the foot, in the depression distal and inferior to the medial malleolus, the midpoint.

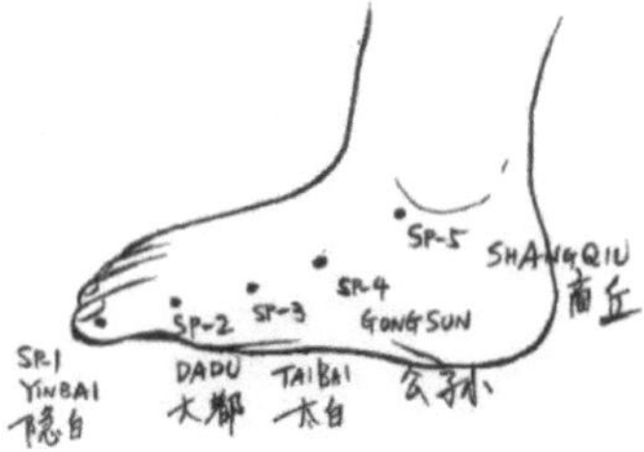

SP-6 (Sanyinjiao 三阴交)

Indications

Abdominal pain and distension, edema, irregular menstruation, metrorrhagia, metrostaxis, leukorrhea, amenorrhea, insomnia, hypertension, muscular atrophy, paralysis of the lower extremities, dizziness, hernia, pain in the external genitalia.

Location

3 cun directly above the tip of medial malleolus, in the depression near the posterior border of the tibia.

SP-7 (Lougu 漏谷)

Indications

Abdominal pain and distension, borborygmus, numbness, paralysis of the lower limbs.

Location

6 cun above the tip of the medial malleolus, og 3 cun superior to SP-6 (Sanyinjiao 三阴交), in a depression posterior.

SP-8 (Diji 地机)

- **Xi-Cleft point of the Spleen channel.**

Indications

Abdominal pain, diarrhea, edema, irregular mensteruation, dysmenorrhea, dysuria, paralysis of the lower limbs.

Location

3 cun below SP-9 (Yinlingquan 阴陵泉), on the line connecting the tip of the medial malleolus.

SP-9 (Yinlingquan 阴陵泉)

- **He-Sea point of the Spleen channel.**

Indications

Abdominal pain and distension, diarrhea, constipation, dysentery, edema, dysuria, jaundice, pain in the knee, pain in the external genitalia.

Location

On the medial side of the lower leg, in a depression posterior and inferior to the medial condyle to the tibia.

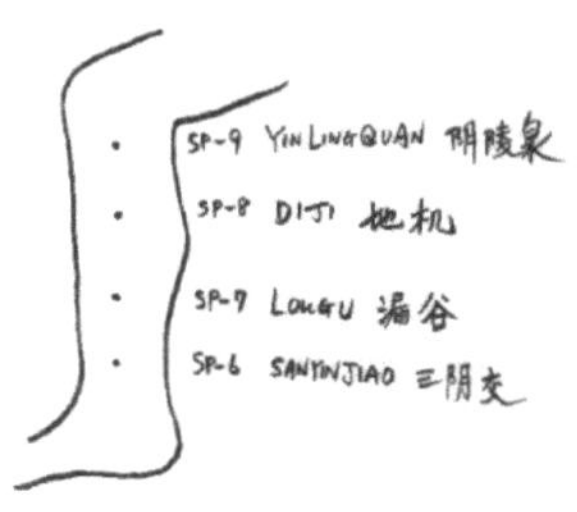

SP-10 (Xuehai 血海)

- **Sea of Blood.**

Indications

Irregular menstruation, dysmenorrhea, amenorrhea, exzema, urticaria, pain of the knee joint.

Location

When the knee is flexed, 2 cun above medial border of the patella, directly above SP-9 (Yinlingquan 阴陵泉).

When the knee is flexed, put the palm on the upper border of the patella with four fingers directed upward, and the thumb forming an angle of 45 degrees with the index finger. The point is where the tip of the thumb.

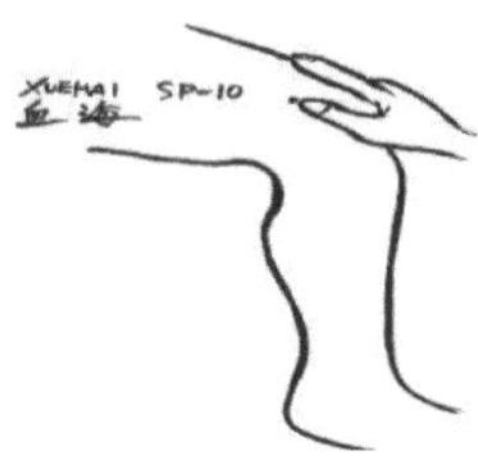

SP-11 (Jimen 箕门)

Indications

Dysuria, enuresis, muscular atrophy, paralysis of the lower extremities.

Location

On the medial side of the thigh, 6 cun above SP-10 (Xuehai 血海).

SP-12 (Chongmen 冲门)

Indications

Lower abdominal pain, hernia, dysuria, leukorrhagia, irregular menstruation.

Location

6 cun above SP-10 (Xuehai 血海), 3.5 cun lateral to the midpoint of the upper border of the symphysis pubis.

SP-13 (Fushe 府舍)

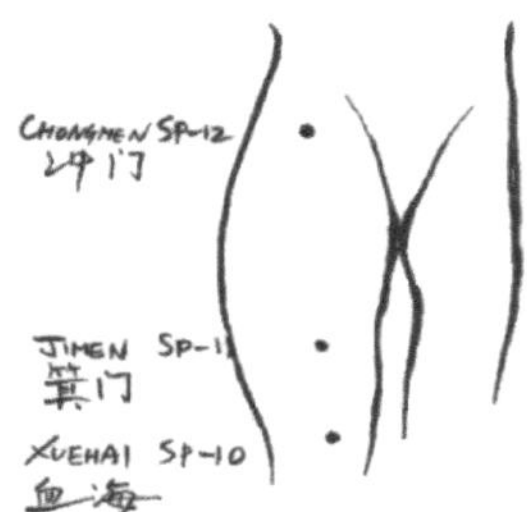

Indications

Lower abdominal pain, hernia.

Location

On the lower abdomen, 0.7 cun superior to SP-12 (Chongmen 冲门), 4 cun lateral to the midline.

SP-14 (Fujie 腹結)

Indications

Abdominal distension, hernia, diarrhea, constipation.

Location

On the lower abdomen, 3 cun above SP-13 (Fushe 府舍).

SP-15 (Daheng 大橫)

Indications

Abdominal pain and distension, diarrhea, dysentery, constipation.

Location

On the abdomen, 4 cun lateral to the center of the umbilicus.

SP-16 (Fuai 腹哀)

Indications

Abdominal pain, constipation, sysentery.

Location

On the abdomen, 3 cun above the umbilicus, 4 cun lateral to the anterior midline.

SP-17 (Shidou 食窦)

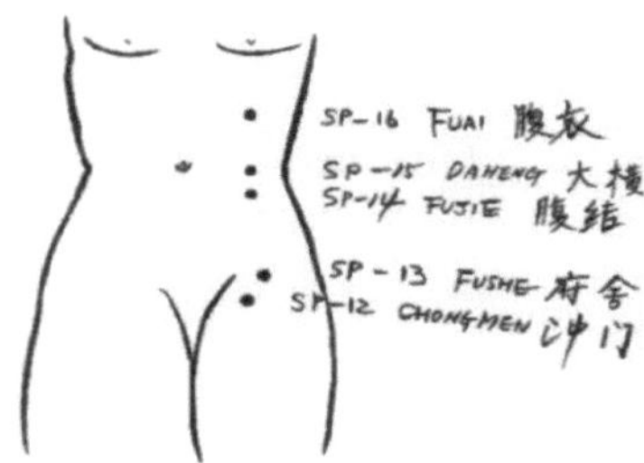

Indications

Pain in the chest and hypochondriac region.

Location

On the lateral side of the chest, in the fifth intercostal space, 6 cun lateral to the anterior midline.

SP-18 (Tianxi 天溪)

Indications

Pain in the chest and hypochondriac region, cough, hiccup, mastitis.

Location

On the lateral side of the chest, in the fourth intercostal space, 6 cun lateral to the anterior midline.

SP-19 (Xiongxiang 胸乡)

Indications

Pain in the chest and hypochondriac region.

Location

On the lateral side of the chest, in the third intercostal space, 6 cun lateral to the anterior midline.

SP-20 (Zourong 周荣)

Indications

Pin in the chest and hypochondriac region, cough, hiccup.

Location

On the lateral side of the chest, in the second intercostal space, 6 cun lateral to the midline.

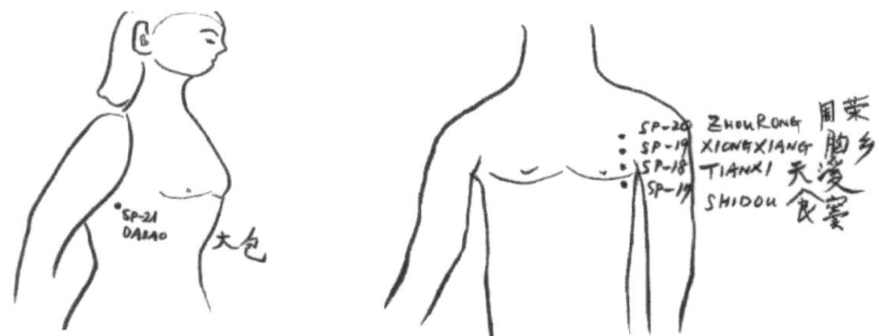

SP-21 (Dabao 大包)

- **Great Luo-Connecting point of the Spleen.**

Indications

Pain in the chest and hypochondriac, cough, asthma, general pain and flaccidity of the extremities.

Location

On the lateral side of the chest, in the middle axillary line, in the sixth intercostal space.

V. The Heart Channel of Hand-Taiyang
手阴心经经穴

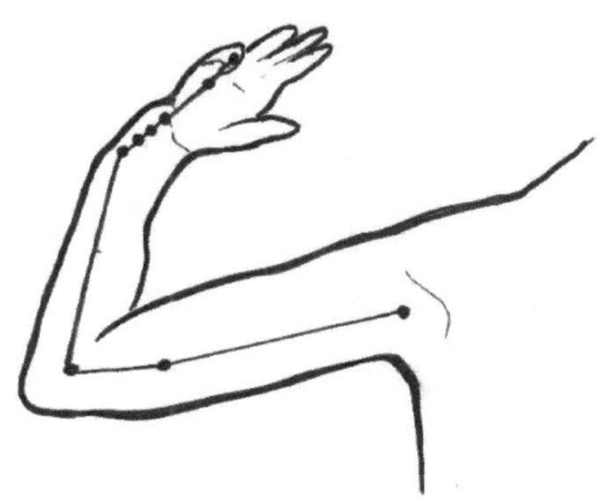

Starts in the armpit, passing through the forearm to the pisiform region proximal to the palm, then follows to the tip of the little finger. It contains 9 different acupoints.

HT-1 (Jiquan 极泉)

Indications

Angina pectoris, chest distress, hypochondriac and costal pain, dry mouth, yellowish eyes, cold pain in the arm.

Location

When raise the arm, the point in the depression at the centre of the axilla

HT-2 (Qingling 青灵)

Indications

Pain in cardiac and hypochondriac regions, shoulder and arm.

Location

3 cun above the medial end of the transverse cubital crease, on the line connecting HT-1 (Jiquan 极泉) and HT-3 (Shaohai 少海).

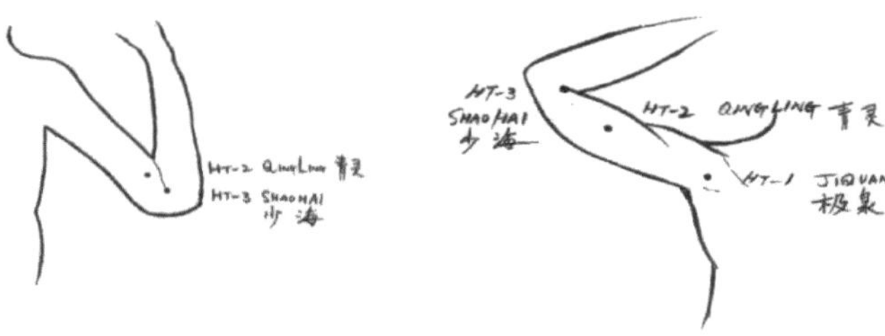

HT-3 (Shaohai 少海)

- **He-Sea point of the Heart channel.**

Indications

Cardiac pain, mania, epilepsy, numbness of arm and hand, pain in the axilla, tremor of hand, scrofula, headache, toothache.

Location

When the elbow is flexed, at the midpoint of the line jointing the medial end of the transverse cubital crease.

HT-4 (Lingdao 灵道)

Indications

Angina pectoris, palpitation, spasmodic pain of the elbow and arm, aphasia, sorrow and fright.

Location

On the palm side of the forearm, 1.5 cun above
the transverse crease of the wrist.

HT-5 (Tongli 通里)

- **Luo-Connecting point of the Heart channel.**

Indications

Palpitation, dizziness, sudden loss of voice,
aphasia due to stiff tongue, pain in the wrist and
arm.

Location

On the palm side of the forearm, 1 cun above the
transverse crease of the wrist.

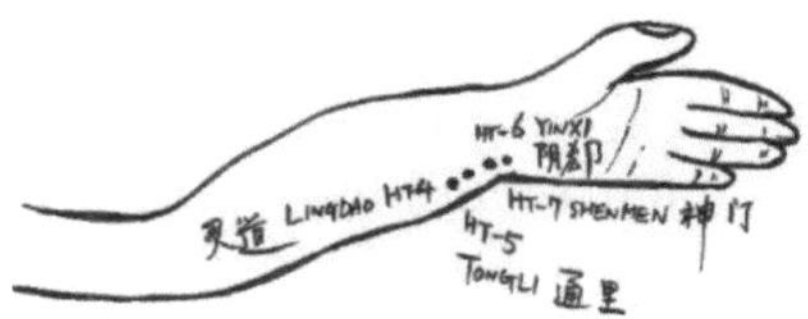

HT-6 (Yinxi 阴郄)

- **Xi-Cleft point of the Heart channel.**

Indications

Angina pectoris, palpitation, epistaxis, sudden
loss of voice, epistaxis, blurring of vision.

Location

On the palmer side of the forearm, 0.5 cun above
the transverse crease of the wrist.

HT-7 (Shenmen 神门)

- **Yuan-Source of the Heart channel.**

Indications

68

Angina pectoris, Insomnia, palpitation, mania, epilepsy, hypochondriac pain, wrist pain, finger numbness, dementia.

Location

At the ulnar end of the transverse crease of the wrist, on the radial side of flexor carpi ulnaris, in the depression at the proximal border of the pisiform bone.

HT-8 (Shaofu 少府)

Indications

Palpitation, chest pain, dysuria, enuresis, spasmodic pain of the little finger, pruritus of the external genitalia.

Location

On the palm, in the depression between the fourth and fifth metacarpal bones.
When a fist is made, the point is on where the tip of the little finger rests.

HT-9 (Shaochong 少冲)

* **Jing-Well point**

Indications

Palpitation, angina pectoris, mania, loss of consciousness, febrile disease, hypochondriac pain.

Location

On the radial side of the little finger, 0.1 cun beside the corner of the nail.

VI. The Small Intestine Channel of Hand-Taiyang 手太阳小肠经经穴

Starts from the ulnar side of the tip of the little finger and follows the ulnar side of the dorsum of the hand to the wrist, passing through the arm to the shoulder blade to the neck, then up to the eye and across to the ear. It contains 19 different acupoints.

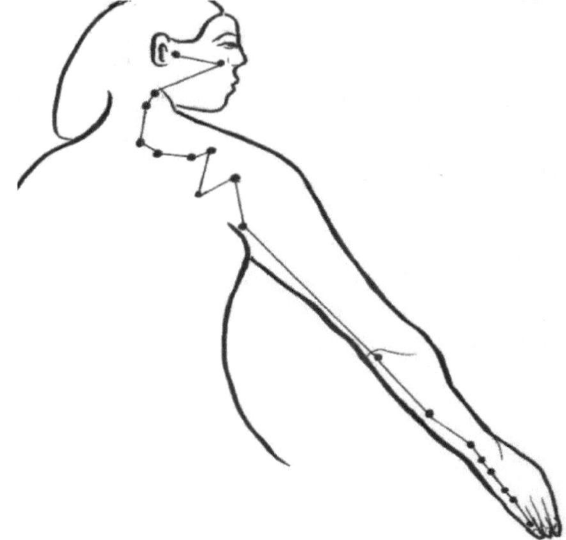

SI-1 (Shaoze 少泽)

- **Jing-Well point.**

Indications

> Apoplexy, loss of consciousness, cataract, tinnitus, deafness, sore throat, breast abscess, headache, febrile diseases.

Location

On the ulnar side of the little finger, 0.1 un from the corner of the nail.

SI-2 (Qiangu 前谷)

Indications

Headache, numbness of the fingers, tinnitus, deafness.

Location

When a loose fist is made, the point on the ulnar end of the crease, side of the 5th metacarpophalangeal joint.

SI-3 (Houxi 后溪)

Indications

Tinnitus, deafness, sore throat, mania, epilepsy, stiff neck, numbness of the fingers, pain in the shoulder and elbow, febrile diseases.

Location

When a loose fist is made, the point on the ulnar side of the hand, at the end of the transverse crease proximal to the fifth metacarpophalangeal joint.

SI-4 (Wangu 腕骨)

- **Yuan-Source point of the Small Intestine Channel.**

Indications

Tinnitus, deafness, numbness of fingers, febrile disease, jaundice, cataract, pain and stiffness of neck.

Location

On the ulnar side of the hand, in the depression between the base of the fifth metacarpal bone and the triquetral bone.

SI-5 (Yanggu 阳谷)

Indications

Headache, tinnitus, deafness, mania, epilepsy, swelling and pain of the eyes, febrile disease, pain of the hand and wrist, swelling of the neck.

Location

At the ulnar side of the wrist, in the depression between styloid process of the ulna and the triquetral bone.

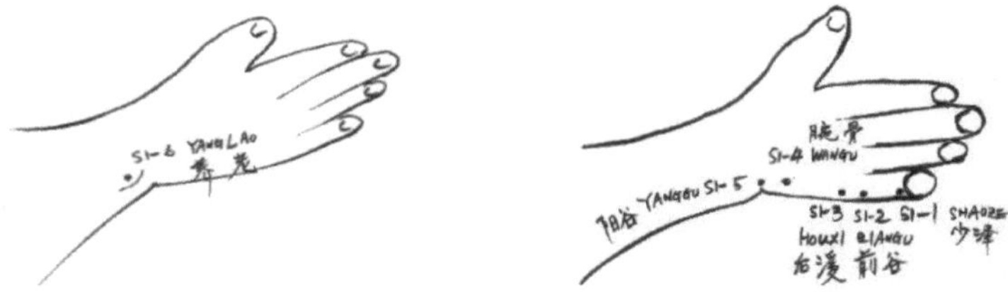

SI-6 (Yanglao 养老)

- **Xi-Cleft point of the Small Intestine channel.**

Indications

Blurred vision, pain in the shoulder, back, elbow and arm.

Location

With the palm facing downward, put a fingertip on the highest spot of the head of ulna, in a depression under the finger, on the radial side of the styloid process of the ulna.

SI-7 (Zhizheng 支正)

- **Luo-connecting point of the Small Intestine channel. Indications.**

Headache, dizziness, depressive psychosis, mania, febrile diseases, pain in the elbow, arm and fingers.

Location

On the line connecting SI-6 (Yanglao 养老) and SI-8(Xiaohai 小海), 5 cun proximal to the dorsal crease of the wrist.

SI-8(Xiaohai 小海)

- **He-Sea point of the Small Intestine channel.**

Indications

Headache, dizziness, tinnitus, deafness, epilepsy, pain in the shoulder, arm and elbow.

Location

When the elbow is flexed, in the depression between the olecranon of the ulna and the tip of the medial epicondyle of the humerus.

SI-9 (Jianzhen 肩贞)

Indications

Numbness of the upper limbs, tinnitus and deafness, inability to raise shoulder, pain in the scapular region.

Location

On the shoulder, posterior and inferior to the shoulder joint. 1 cun above the posterior end of the axillary fold.

SI-10 (Naoshu 臑俞)

Indications

Pain in the shoulder and scrofula.

Location

On the shoulder, above the posterior end of the axillary fold, in the depression below the lower border of the scapular spine.

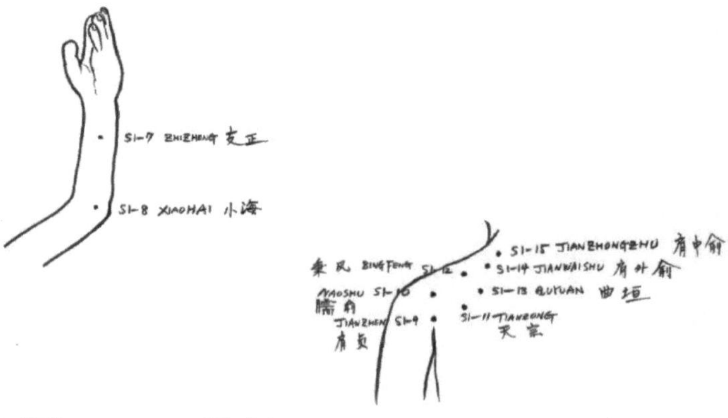

SI-11 (Tianzong 天宗)

Indications

Pain in the scapular region, cough asthma, breast abscess.

Location

On the scapula, in the depression of the center of the subscapular fossa, at the same level of the fourth thoracic vertebra.

SI-12 (Bingfeng 秉风)

Indications

Pain in the scapular region, inability to raise shoulder, numbness of upper limbs.

Location

On the scapra, in the centre of the suprascapular fossa, directly above SI-11 (Tianzong 天宗), in a dipression found when the arm is lifted.

SI-13 (Quyuan 曲垣)

Indications

Pain in the scapular region.

Location

On the chest, in the fourth intercostal space, at the corner of the nipple, 4 cun lateral to the anterior midline.

SI-14 (Jianwaishu 肩外俞)

Indications

Aching pain in the shoulder and back, pain and stiffness of neck, cough, asthma.

Location

3 cun lateral to the lower border of the spinous process of the 1st thoracic vertebra.

SI-15 (Jianzhongshu 肩中俞)

Indications

Cough, asthma, stiff neck, headache, aching pain in the shoulder and back.

Location

2 cun lateral to DU-14 (Dazhui 大椎).

SI-16 (Tianchuang 天窗)

Indications

Tinnitus, deafness, pain and stiffness of neck, sore throat, loss of voice.

Location

Posterior border of the sternocleido-mastoid muscle level with the laryngeal prominence.

SI-17 (Tianrong 天容)

Indications

Tinnitus, deafness, sore throat, pain and swelling of the neck, goiter.

Location

Posterior to the angle of the mandible, in the depression on the anterior border of the sternocleidomastoid muscle.

SI-18 (Quanliao 颧髎)

Indications

Facial paralysis, twitching of eyelids, toothache, pain and swelling in the face.

Location

Directly below the outer canthus, in the depression of the lower border of the zygomatic bone.

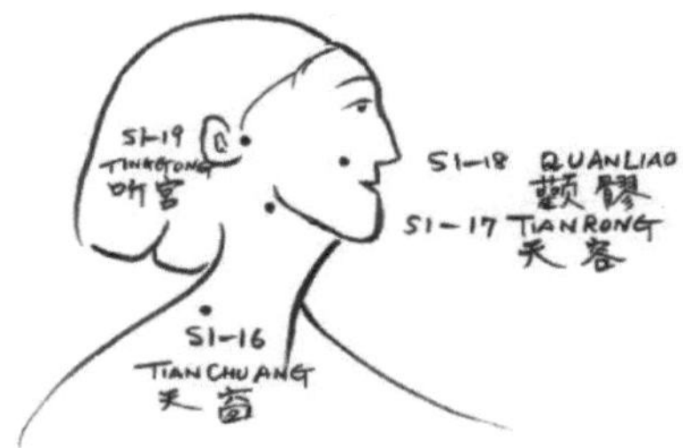

SI-19 (Tinggong 听宫)

Indications

Tinnitus, deafness, toothache, motor impairment of the mandibular.

Location

In the depression formed when the mouth is open. Anterior to the tragus and posterior to the condyloid process of the mandible

VII. The Bladder channel of Foot-Taiyang
足太阳膀胱经经穴

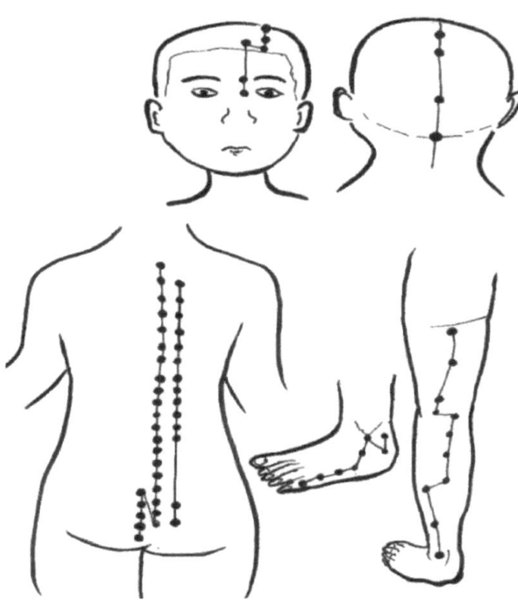

Starts in the eye and ascending to the forehead and over the top of the skull. It splits below the hairline in back. One branch passes through down the shoulder blade and down to the middle of the low back. The other one passes downward to the outside of the spine through down the back of the leg to the heel. It contains 67 different acupuncture points.

BL-1 (Jingming 睛明)
Indications

Redness, swelling and pain of eyes, blurred vision, dizziness, nearsightedness, color blindness.

Location

On the closed eye, in the depression slightly above, 0.1 cun lateral and superior to the inner canthus.

BL-2 (Zanzhu 攒竹)

Indications

Headache, blurred vision, pain and swelling of the eyes, twitching of eyelids, glaucoma.

Location

On the face, directly above BL-1 (Jingming 睛明), in the depression on the medial end of the eyebrow.

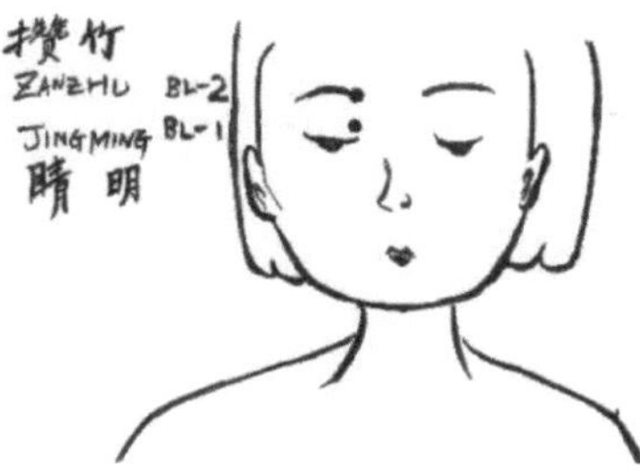

BL-3 (Meichong 眉冲)

Indications

Headache, epilepsy, nasal obstruction.

Location

On the head, directly above BL-2 (Zanzhu 攒竹), 0.5 cun above the anterior hairline.

BL-4 (Qucha 曲差)

Indications

Headache, nasal obstruction, epitasis, blurring vision.

Location

On the head, 0.5 cun above the anterior hairline, 1.5 cun lateral to the midline.

BL-5 (Wuchu 五处)

Indications

Headache, blurring vision, epilepsy, convulsion.

Location

On the head, 1 cun directly above the midway of the anterior hairline, 1.5 cun lateral to the anterior midline.

BL-6 (Chengguang 承光)

Indications

Headache, nasal obstruction, blurring vision.

Location

On the head, 2.5 cun directly above the midway of the anterior hairline, 1.5 cun lateral to the anterior midline.

BL-7 (Tongtian 通天)

Indications

Headache, epistaxis, nasal obstruction, giddiness, rhinorrhea.

Location

On the head, 4 cun directly above the midway of the anterior hairline, 1.5 cun lateral to the anterior midline.

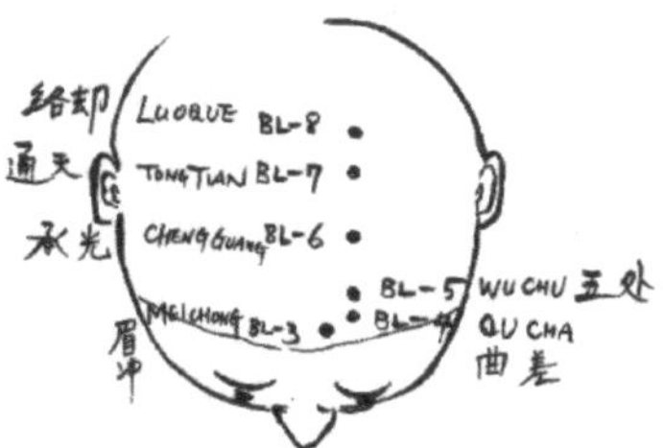

BL-8 (Louque 络却)

Indications

Dizziness, blurring of vision, tinnitus, mania.

Location

On the head, 5.5 cun directly above the midway of the anterior hairline, 1.5 cun lateral to the anterior midline.

BL-9 (Yuzhen 玉枕)

Indications

Headache, neck pain, dizziness, nasal obstruction, ophthalmalgia.

Location

On the occiput, 2.5 cun directly above the midpoint of the posterior hairline and 1.3 cun lateral to the midline, in the depression on the level of the upper border of the external occipital protuberance.

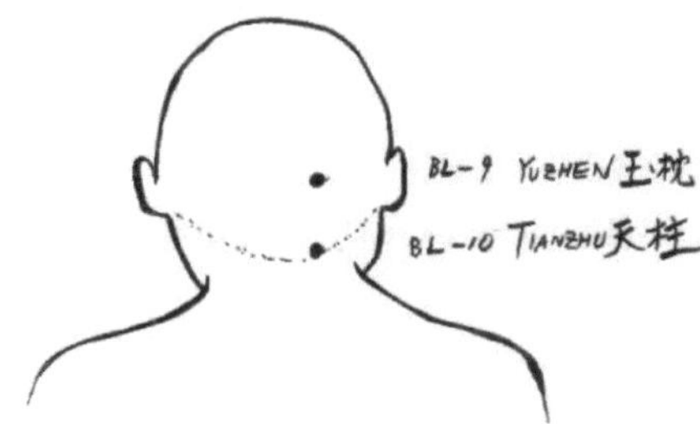

BL-10 (Tianzhu 天柱)

Indications

Headache, Stiff neck, pain in the shoulder and back, epilepsy, nasal obstruction, depression, mania.

Location

1.3 cun lateral to the midpoint of the posterior hairline, in the depression on the lateral border of the trapezius muscle.

BL-11 (Dazhu 大杼)

- **Point of the Sea of Blood.**

Indications

Pain the shoulder and back, stiff neck, nasal obstruction, headache, cough, sore throat, fever.

Location

On the back, below the spinous process of the first thoracic vertebra (T1), 1.5 cun lateral to the posterior midline.

BL-12 (Fengmen 风门)

Indications

Common cold, cough, headache, fever, stiff neck, running nose.

Location

On the back, below the spinous process of the second thoracic vertebra (T2), 1.5 cun lateral to the posterior midline.

BL-13 (Feishu 肺俞)

- **Back-Shu point of the Lung.**

Indications

Chest pain, cough, asthma, tidal fever, night sweating, nasal obstruction.

Location

On the back, below the spinous process of the third thoracic vertebra (T3), 1.5 cun lateral to the posterior midline.

BL-14 (Jueyinshu 厥阴俞)

- **Back-Shu point of the Pericardium.**

Indications

Palpitation, angina pectoris, cough, vomiting, oppression.

Location

On the back, below the spinous process of the fourth thoracic vertebra (T4), 1.5 cun lateral to the posterior midline.

BL-15 (Xinshu 心俞)

- **Back-Shu point of the Heart.**

Indications

Angina pectoris, palpitation, cough, epilepsy, insomnia, mania, night sweating.

Location

On the back, below the spinous process of the fifth thoracic vertebra (T5), 1.5 cun lateral to the posterior midline.

BL-16 (Dushu 督俞)

Indications

Angina pectoris, abdominal pain, chest oppression, asthma, alternate chills and fever.

Location

On the back, below the spinous process of the sixth thoracic vertebra (T6), 1.5 cun lateral to the posterior midline.

BL-17 (Geshu 膈俞)

Indications

Vomiting, hiccup, asthma, cough, spitting blood, afternoon fever, night sweating.

Location

82

On the back, below the spinous process of the seventh thoracic vertebra (T7), 1.5 cun lateral to the posterior midline.

BL-18 (Ganshu 肝俞)

- **Back-Shu point of the Liver.**

Indications

Jaundice, hypochondriac pain, dizziness, blurred vision, redness of the eye, epilepsy, mania, depression.

Location

On the back, below the spinous process of the ninth thoracic vertebra (T9), 1.5 cun lateral to the posterior midline.

BL-19 (Danshu 胆俞)

- **Back-Shu point of the Gall Bladder.**

Indications

Jaundice, bitter taste in the mouth, hypochondriac pain, lung tuberculosis, tidal fever.

Location

On the back, below the spinous process of the tenth thoracic vertebra (T10), 1.5 cun lateral to the posterior midline.

BL-20 (Pishu 脾俞)

- **Back-Shu point of the Spleen.**

Indications

Abdominal pain, jaundice, vomiting, diarrhea, dysentery, edema, pain of back.

Location

On the back, below the spinous process of the eleventh thoracic vertebra (T11), 1.5 cun lateral to the posterior midline.

BL-21 (Weishu 胃俞)

- **Back-Shu point of the Stomach.**

Indications

Stomachache, vomiting, hiccup, abdominal distension, borborygmus, pain in the chest and back.

Location

On the back, below the spinous process of the twelfth thoracic vertebra (T12), 1.5 cun lateral to the posterior midline.

BL-22 (Sanjiaoshu 三焦俞)

- **Back-Shu point of the Sanjiao.**

Indications

Borborygmus, abdominal distension, diarrhea, dysentery, edema, stiffness of the lower back.

Location

On the lower back, below the spinous process of the first lumbar vertebra (L1), 1.5 cun lateral to the posterior midline.

BL-23 (Shenshu 肾俞)

- **Back-Shu point of the Kidneys.**

Indications

Seminal emission, impotence, enuresis, irregular menstruation, leukorrhea, tinnitus, deafness, edema, asthma.

84

Location

On the lower back, below the spinous process of the second lumbar vertebra (L2), 1.5 cun lateral to the posterior midline.

BL-24 (Qihaishu 气海俞)

- **Sea of Qi Shu.**

Indications

Low back pain, abdominal distension, dysmenorrhea, lumbago, hemorrhoids.

Location

On the lower back, below the spinous process of the third lumbar vertebra (L3), 1.5 cun lateral to the posterior midline.

BL-25 (Dachangshu 大肠俞)

- **Large Intestine Shu**

Indications

Abdominal distension, borborygmus, diarrhea, constipation, dysentery, lumbago, sciatica, numbness and motor impairment of the lower extremities.

Location

On the lower back, below the spinous process of the fouth lumbar vertebra (L4), 1.5 cun lateral to the posterior midline.

BL-26 (Guanyuanshu 关元俞)

- **Gate of the Origin Shu.**

Indications

Abdominal distension, diarrhea, enuresis, lumbago, sciatica, frequent urination.

Location

On the lower back, below the spinous process of the fifth lumbar vertebra (L5), 1.5 cun lateral to the posterior midline.

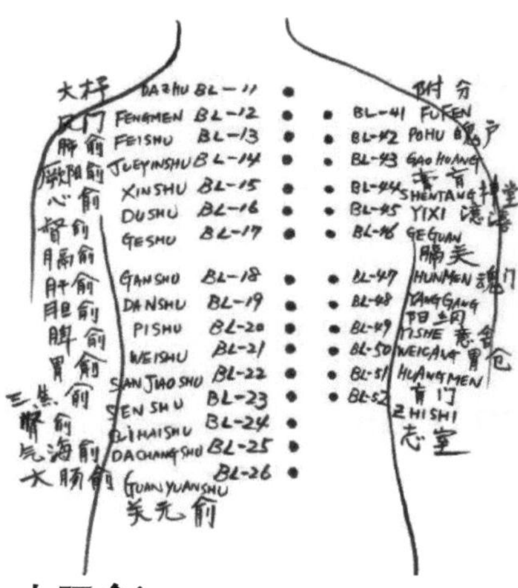

BL-27 (Xiaochangshu 小肠俞)

- **Back-Shu point of the Small Intestine.**

Indications

Abdominal distension, diarrhea, dysentery, enuresis, hematuria, leukorrhea, lumbago, lower back pain, sciatica.

Location

On the sacrum, 1.5 cun lateral to the midline, at the level of the first posterior sacral foramen.

BL-28 (Pangguangshu 膀胱俞)

- **Back-Shu point of the Bladder.**

Indications

Retention of urine, dysuria, enuresis, diarrhea, constipation, pain of the lower back.

Location

On the sacrum, 1.5 cun lateral to the midline, at the level of the second posterior sacral foramen.

BL-29 (Zhonglushu 中膂)

- **Mid-Spine Shu.**

Indications

Hernia, diarrhea, stiffness and pain of the lower back.

Location

On the sacrum, 1.5 cun lateral to the midline, at the level of the third posterior sacral foramen.

BL-30 (Baihuanshu 白环俞)

- **White Ring Shu.**

Indications

Enuresis, hernia, seminal emission, irregular menstruation, constipation, dysuria, prolapse of the rectum.

Location

On the sacrum, 1.5 cun lateral to the midline, at the level of the fourth posterior sacral foramen.

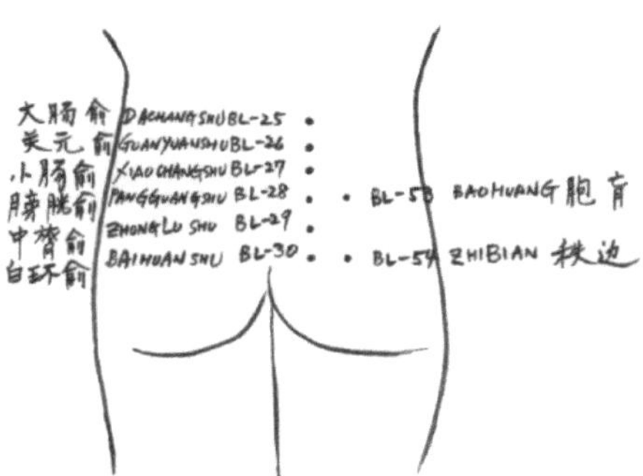

BL-31 (Shangliao 上髎)

Indications

Low back pain, dysuria, irregular menstruation, leukorrhea, impotence.

Location

On the sacrum, first posterior sacral foramen.

BL-32 (Ciliao 次髎)

Indications

Irregular menstruation, dysmenorrhea, hernia, dysuria, leukorrhea, seminal emission, muscular atrophy, numbness and motor impairment of the lower extremities.

Location

On the sacrum, second posterior sacral foramen.

BL-33 (Zhongliao 中髎)

Indications

Constipation, diarrhea, low back pain, irregular menstruation, leukorrhea, dysuria.

Location

On the sacrum, third posterior sacral foramen.

BL-34 (Xialiao 下髎)

Indications

Abdominal pain, constipation, leukorrhea, irregular menstruation, low back pain.

Location

On the sacrum, fourth posterior sacral foramen.

BL-35 (Huiyang 会阳)

Indications

Hemorrhoids, diarrhea, leukorrhea, hematochezia.

Location

0.5 cun lateral to the tip of the coccyx.

BL-36 (Chengfu 承扶)

Indications

Hemorrhoids, constipation, pain in the lower back and gluteal region, motor impairment of the lower extremities.

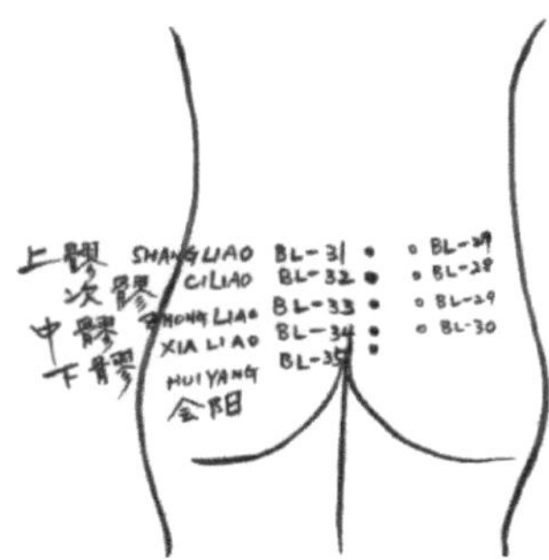

Location

On the midpoint of the transverse gluteal fold, the point in the middle of the back of the thigh.

BL-37 (Yinmen 殷门)

Indications

Hemiplegia, flaccidity and numbness of the lower extremities, muscular atrophy.

Location

On the back of the thigh, 6 cun directly below BL-36 (Chengfu 承扶).

BL-38 (Fuxi 浮郄)

Indications

Numbness of the gluteal and femoral regions, contracture of the tendons in the popliteal fossa.

Location

On the back of the knee, 1 cun above BL-39 (Weiyang 委阳), on the medial side of the tendon of biceps femoris on the lateral side of the popliteal fossa.

BL-39 (Weiyang 委阳)

- **Lower He-Sea point of the Sanjiao.**

Indications

Abdominal fullness, dysuria, stiffness and pain of the lower back, edema, dysuria, cramp of the legs and foot.

Location

On the back of the knee, at the lateral end of the popliteal crease, on the medial border of the tendon of biceps femoris.

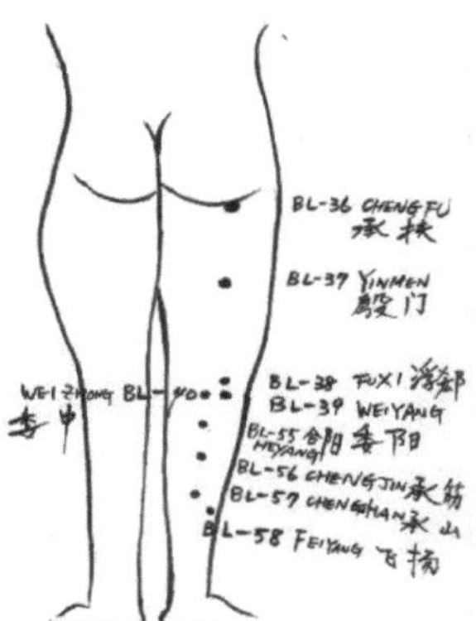

BL-40 (Weizhong 委中)

- **He-Sea point of the Bladder channel.**

Indications

Lumbago, dysuria, enuresis, abdominal pain, vomiting, diarrhea, vomiting, diarrhea, flaccidity and obstruction syndromes of lower limbs.

Location

On the back of the knee, on the midpoint of the transverse crease of the popliteal fossa.

BL-41 (Fufen 附分)

Indications

Pain and stiffness of the shoulder, back and neck, numbness of the elbow and arm.

Location

On the back, below the spinous process of the second thoracic vertebra (T2), 3 cun lateral to the midline and level with BL-12 (Fengmen 风门).

BL-42 (Pohu 魄户)

Indications

Cough, asthma, pain the shoulder and back, hemoptysis, pulmonary tuberculosis.

Location

On the back, below the spinous process of the third thoracic vertebra (T3), 3 cun lateral to the midline and level with BL-13 (Feishu 肺俞).

BL-43 (Gaohuangshu 膏肓俞)

Indications

Pulmonary tuberculosis, cough, asthma, hemoptysis, insomnia, nocturnal emission.

Location

On the back, below the spinous process of the fourth thoracic vertebra (T4), 3 cun lateral to the midline and level with BL-14 (Jueyinshu 厥阴俞).

BL-44 (Shentang 神堂)

Indications

Cardiac pain, palpitation, asthma, cough, pain and stiffness of the back.

Location

On the back, below the spinous process of the fifth thoracic vertebra (T5), 3 cun lateral to the midline and level with BL-15 (Xinshu 心俞).

BL-45 (Yixi 噫嘻)

Indications

Cough, asthma, pain of the shoulder and neck.

Location

On the back, below the spinous process of the sixth thoracic vertebra (T6), 3 cun lateral to the midline and level with BL-16 (Dushu 督俞).

BL-46 (Geguan 膈关)

Indications

Vomiting, belching, hiccup, pain in the spine and back, chest oppression.

Location

On the back, below the spinous process of the seventh thoracic vertebra (T7), 3 cun lateral to the midline and level with BL-17 (Geshu 膈俞).

BL-47 (Hunmen 魂门)

Indications

Pain in the chest and hypochondriac region, vomiting, diarrhea, back pain.

Location

On the back, below the spinous process of the ninth thoracic vertebra (T9), 3 cun lateral to the midline and level with BL-18 (Ganshu 肝俞).

BL-48 (Yanggang 阳刚)

Indications

Abdominal pain, borborygmus, diarrhea, jaundice, diabetes, pain in hypochondriac.

Location

On the back, below the spinous process of the tenth thoracic vertebra (T10), 3 cun lateral to the midline and level with BL-19 (Danshu 胆俞).

BL-49 (Yishe 意舍)

Indications

Abdominal distension, vomiting, diarrhea, borborygmus, difficulty in swallowing.

Location

On the back, below the spinous process of the eleventh thoracic vertebra (T11), 3 cun lateral to the midline and level with BL-20 (Pishu 脾俞).

BL-50 (Weicang 胃仓)

Indications

Abdominal distension, pain in the epigastric region and back.

Location

On the back, below the spinous process of the twelfth thoracic vertebra (T12), 3 cun lateral to the midline and level with BL-21 (Weishu 胃俞).

BL-51 (Huangmen 肓门)

Indications

Abdominal pain, constipation.

Location

On the lower back, below the spinous process of the first lumber vertebra (L1), 3 cun lateral to the midline and level with BL-22 (Sanjiaoshu 三焦俞).

BL-52 (Zhishi 志室)

Indications

Seminal emission, dysuria, edema, pain in the back and knee, irregular menstruation.

Location

On the lower back, below the spinous process of the second lumber vertebra (L2), 3 cun lateral to the midline and level with BL-23 (Shenshu 肾俞).

BL-53 (Baohuang 包肓)

Indications

Abdominal distension, borborygmus, pain in the lower back.

Location

On the buttock, 3 cun lateral to the midline, level with the second posterior sacral foramen.

BL-54 (Zhibian 秩边)

Indications

Motor impairment of the lower extremities, dysuria, constipation, hemorrhoids, muscular atrophy.

Location

On the buttock, 3 cun lateral to the midline, level with the fourth posterior sacral foramen.

BL-55 (Heyang 合阳)

Indications

Low back pain, paralysis of the lower extremities.

Location

On the posterior side of the leg, 2 cun directly below to BL-40 (Weizhong 委中).

BL-56 (Chengjin 承筋)

Indications

Hemorrhoids, lower back pain, spasm of gastrocnemius.

Location

On the lower leg, 5 cun below BL-40 (Weizhong 委中), in the centre of the belly of gastrocnemius muscle.

BL-57 (Chengshan 承山)

Indications

Spasm of gastrocnemius, hemorrhoids, constipation, prolapse of rectum, constipation, beriberi.

Location

On the lower leg, 8 cun below BL-40 (Weizhong 委中), midway between BL-40 (Weizhong 委中) and BL-60 (Kunlun 昆仑).

BL-58 (Feiyang 飞扬)

- **Luo-connecting point of the Bladder channel.**

Indications

Headache, dizziness, epistaxis, blurring of vision, hemorrhoids, pain in the waist and leg.

Location

On the lower leg, 7 cun directly above BL-60 (Kunlun 昆仑).

BL-59 (Fuyang 跗阳)

Indications

Headache, low back pain, swelling and pain of external malleolus, paralysis of the lower extremities.

Location

On the lower leg, 3 cun directly above BL-60 (Kunlun 昆仑).

BL-60 (Kunlun 昆仑)

Indications

Headache, dizziness, blurring vision, pain and swelling of the heel, low pack pain, epilepsy, epistaxis.

Location

Behind the ankle joint, in the depression between the prominence of the lateral malleolus.

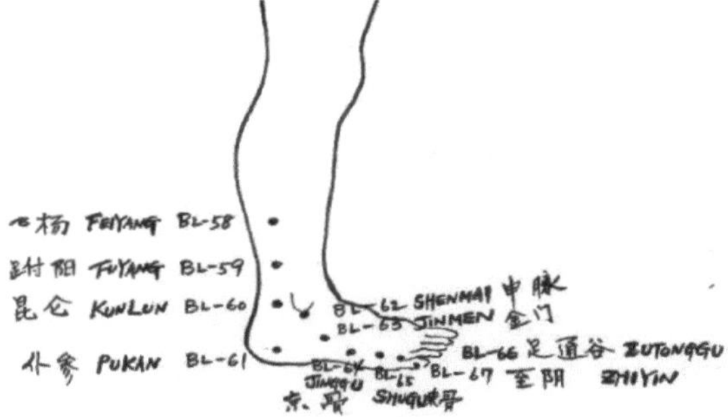

BL-61 (Pucan 仆参)

Indications

Pain in the heel, epilepsy, muscular atrophy, weakness of the lower extremities.

Local

On the lateral side of the foot, directly below BL-60 (Kunlun 昆仑).

BL-62 (Shenmai 申脉)

Indications

Epilepsy, mania, headache, dizziness, insomnia, aching of the leg.

Location

On the lateral side of the foot, directly below the lateral malleolus.

BL-63 (Jinmen 金门)

- **Xi-Cleft point of the Bladder channel.**

Indications

Headache, epilepsy, mania, pain in the external malleolus, flaccidity and motor impairment of lower limbs.

Local

On the lateral side of the foot, in the depression below the cuboid bone which lies between the heel bone and the tuberosity of the 5th metatarsal bone.

BL-64 (Jinggu 京骨)

- **Yuan-Source point of the Bladder channel.**

Indications

Headache, stiffness of neck, pain in the lower back and thigh, epilepsy, cataract.

Location

On the lateral side of the foot, in the depression below the tuberosity of the 5th metatarsal bone.

BL-65 (Shugu 束骨)

Indications

Headache, stiffness of neck, dizziness, manic depression, pain in the lower extremities, blurred vision.

Location

On the lateral side of the foot, posterior to the fifth metatarsal bone.

BL-66 (Zutonggu 足通谷)

Indications

Headache, stiffness of neck, dizziness, manic, depression, epistaxis.

Location

On the lateral side of the foot, anterior to the fifth metatarso-phalangeal bone.

BL-67 (Zhiyin 至阴)

- **Jing-Well point**

Indications

Headache, epistasis, pain of eyes, malposition of fetus, nasal obstruction, dystocia, feverish sensation in the sole.

Location

On the lateral side of the small toe, about 0.1 cun from the corner of the nail.

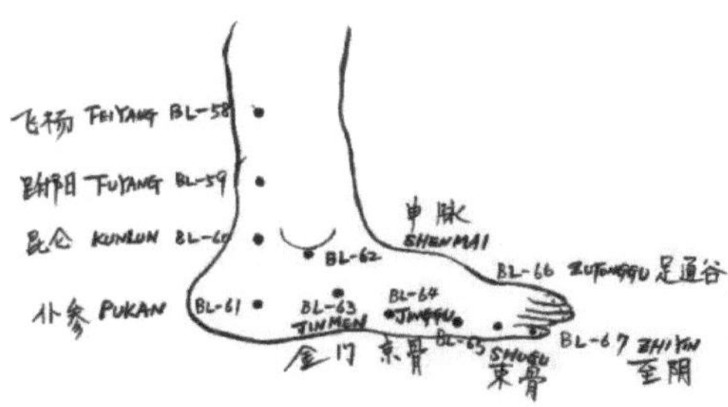

VIII.The Kidney Channel of Foot-Shaoyin
足少阴肾经经穴

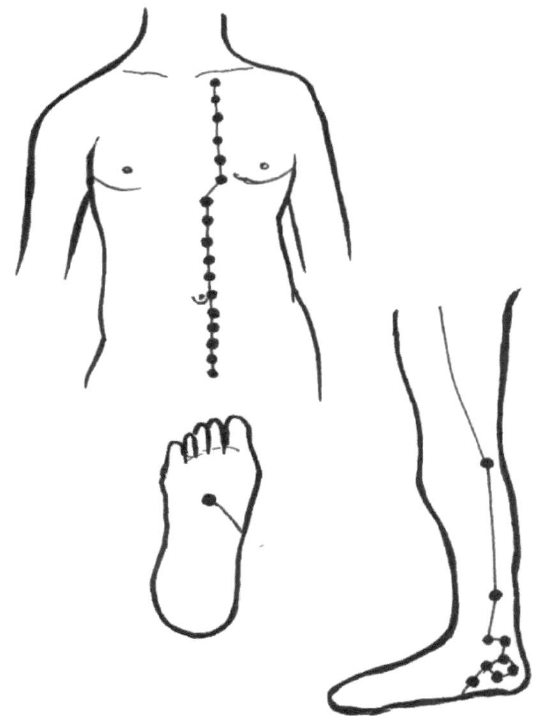

Starts in the arch of the foot and, ascends along the medial side of the leg and to the side of the midline of the abdomen and chest. It contains 27 different acupoints.

KI-1 (Yongquan 涌泉)

- **Jing-Well point**

Indications

Depression, mania, headache, wind stroke, sore throat, dryness of the tongue, feverish soles, dizziness, vertigo, constipation, loss of voice.

Location

On the sole, at the junction of the anterior one-third and posterior two thirds of the sole, between the second and third metatarsal bones.

KI-2 (Rangu 然谷)

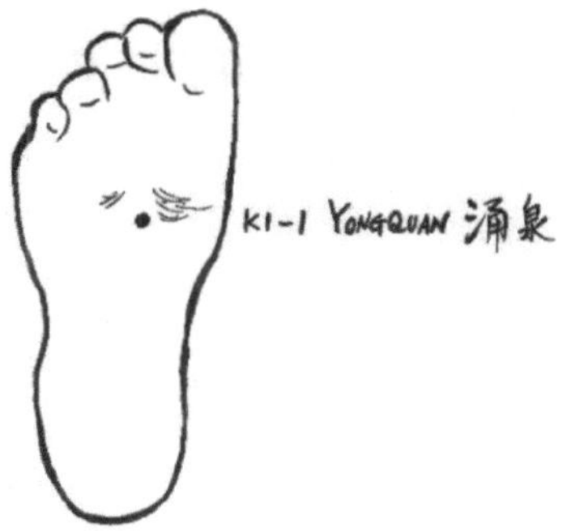

Indications

Headache, dizziness, sore throat, irregular menstruation, leukorrhea, unsmooth urination, seminal emission, pain of the dorsum of foot, hemoptysis.

Location

Anterior and inferior to the medial malleolus, in the depression on the lower border of the tuberosity of the navicular bone.

KI-3 (Taixi 太溪)

- **Yuan-Source of the Kidney channel.**

Indications

Tinnitus, deafness, headache, vertigo, sore throat, toothache, irregular menstruation, cough, asthma, seminal emission, impotence, pain in the heel, insomnia.

Location

On the medial malleolus, in the depression between the prominence of the medial malleolus and the Achilles tendon.

KI-4 (Dazhong 大钟)

- **Luo-Connecting point of the Kidney channel.**

Indications

Asthma, cough, dementia, dysuria, enuresis, frequent urination, pain in the heel, pain of the lower back.

Location

0.5 cun below posterior to KI-3 (Taixi 太溪), on the anterior border of the medial side of the tendon calcaneus.

KI-5 (Shuiquan 水泉)

- **Xi-Cleft point of the Kidney channel.**

Indications

Irregular menstruation, dysmenorrhea, blurred vision, unsmooth urination.

Location

1 cun directly below KI-3 (Taixi 太溪), in the depression of the medial side of the tuberosity of the calcaneum.

KI-6 (Zhaohai 照海)

Indications

Depression, mania, irregular menstruation, dysmenorrhea, insomnia, sore throat, constipation, pain and swelling in the malleolus joint.

Location

1 cun below the prominence of the medial malleolus.

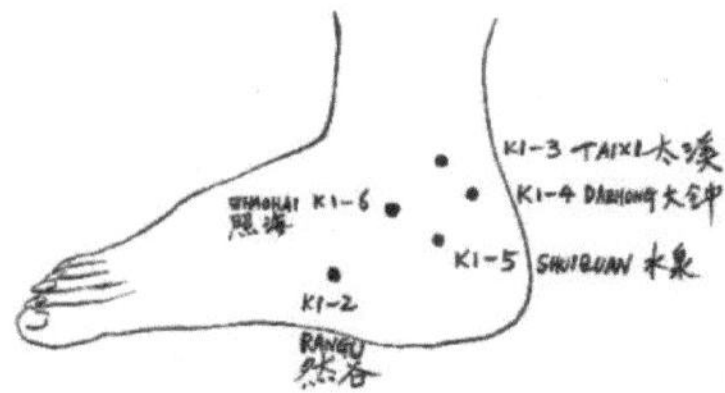

KI-7 (Fuliu 复瘤)

Indications

Edema, Abdominal pain and distension, borborygmus, diarrhea, spontaneous sweating, febrile diseases, flaccidity of lower limbs.

Location

On the medial side of the foot, 2 cun superior to KI-3 (Taixi 太溪) anterior to the Achilles tendon.

KI-8 (Jiaoxin 交信)

Indications

Irregular menstruation, metrorrhagia, dysmenorrhea, constipation, diarrhea, hernia.

Location

On the medial side of the lower leg, 2 cun above KI-3 (Taixi 太溪), 0.5 cun anterior to KI-7 (Fuliu 复瘤).

KI-9 (Zhubin 筑宾)

Indications

Depression, mania, hernia, abdominal pain and distension.

Location

On the medial border of the lower leg, 5 cun superior to KI-3 (Taixi 太溪), on the line connecting KI-3 (Taixi 太溪) and KI-10 (Yingu 阴谷).

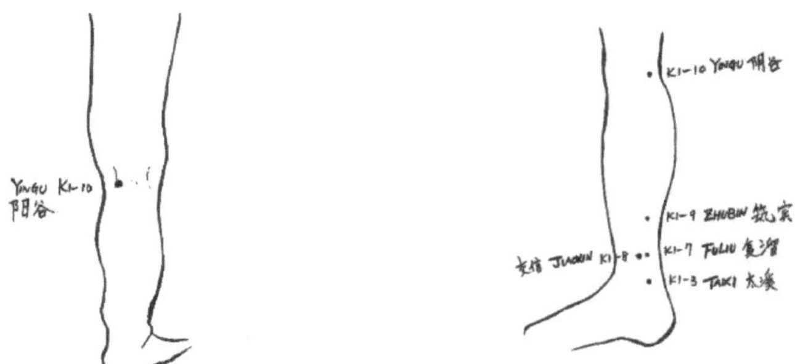

KI-10 (Yingu 阴谷)

- **He-Sea point of the Kidney channel.**

Indications

Hernia, impotence, irregular menstruation, metrorrhagia, pain in the knee, mental disorders.

Location

On the medial end of the popliteal crease, when the knee is flexed, the point is at the medial side of the transverse popliteal fossa.

KI-11 (Henggu 横骨)

Indications

Pain of the lower abdomen, hernia, impotence, enuresis, seminal emission, pain of genitalia.

Location

On the lower abdomen, 5 cun below the umbilicus, 0.5 cun lateral to the anterior midline.

KI-12 (Dahe 大赫)

Indications

Lower abdominal pain, irregular menstruation, leukorrhea, pain in the external genitalia, hernia, seminal emission, impotence.

Location

On the lower abdomen, 4 cun below the umbilicus, 0.5 cun lateral to the anterior midline.

KI-13 (Qixue 气穴)

Indications

Irregular menstruation, dysmenorrhea, dysuria, abdominal pain, diarrhea.

Location

On the lower abdomen, 3 cun below the umbilicus, 0.5 cun lateral to the anterior midline.

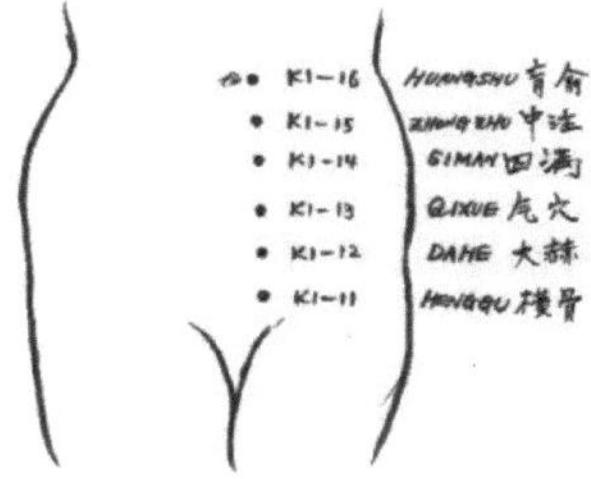

KI-14 (Siman 四满)

Indications

Abdominal pain and distension, diarrhea, irregular menstruation, dysmenorrhea, nocturnal emission.

Location

On the lower abdomen, 2 cun below the umbilicus, 0.5 cun lateral to the anterior midline.

KI-15 (Zhongzhu 中注)

Indications

Irregular menstruation, abdominal pain, constipation.

Location

On the lower abdomen, 1 cun below th umbilicus, 0.5 cun lateral to the anterior midline.

KI-16 (Huangshu 肓俞)

Indications

Abdominal pain and distension, constipation, diarrhea, vomiting.

Location

On the middle abdomen, 0.5 cun lateral to the center of the umbilicus.

KI-17 (Shangqu 商曲)

Indications

Abdominal pain, constipation, diarrhea.

Location

On the upper abdomen, 2 cun above the umbilicus, 0.5 cun lateral to the anterior midline.

KI-18 (Shiguan 石关)

Indications

Abdominal pain, vomiting, constipation.

Location

On the upper abdomen, 3 cun above the umbilicus, 0.5 cun lateral to the anterior midline.

KI-19 (Yindu 阴都)

Indications

Abdominal pain, constipation, Borborygmus, epigastric pain, vomiting.

Location

On the upper abdomen, 4 cun above the umbilicus, 0.5 cun lateral to the anterior midline.

KI-20 (Futonggu 腹通谷)

Indications

Abdominal pain and distension, constipation, vomiting, indigestion.

Location

On the upper abdomen, 5 cun above the umbilicus, 0.5 cun lateral to the anterior midline.

KI-21 (Youmen 幽门)

Indications

Abdominal pain and distension, vomiting, diarrhea, nausea, morning sickness.

Location

On the upper abdomen, 6 cun above the umbilicus, 0.5 cun lateral to the midline.

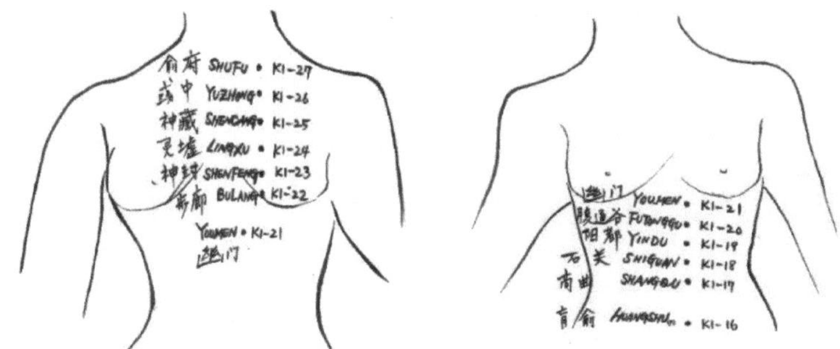

KI-22 (Bulang 步廊)

Indications

Cough, asthma, distension in the chest and hypochondriac region, vomiting, anorexia.

Location

On the chest, in the fifth intercostal space, 2 cun lateral to the midline.

KI-23 (Shenfeng 神封)

Indications

Cough, asthma, fullness in the chest and hypochondriac region.

Location

On the chest, in the fourth intercostal space, and 2 cun lateral to the anterior midline.

KI-24 (Lingxu 灵墟)

Indications

Cough, asthma, fullness in the chest and hypochondriac region.

Location

On the chest, in the third intercostal space, and 2 cun lateral to the anterior midline.

KI-25 (Shencang 神藏)

Indications

Cough, asthma, fullness in the chest and hypochondriac region.

Location

On the chest, in the second intercostal space, and 2 cun lateral to the anterior midline.

KI-26 (Yuzhong 彧中)

Indications

Cough, asthma, fullness in the chest and hypochondriac region, accumulation of phlegm.

Location

On the chest, in the first intercostal space, and 2 cun lateral to the anterior midline.

KI-27 (Shufu 俞府)

Indications

Cough, asthma, chest pain vomiting, anorexia.

Location

On the chest, below the lower border of the clavicle, 2 cun lateral to the midline.

IX. The Pericardium Channel of Hand-Yueyin 手蕨阴心包经经穴

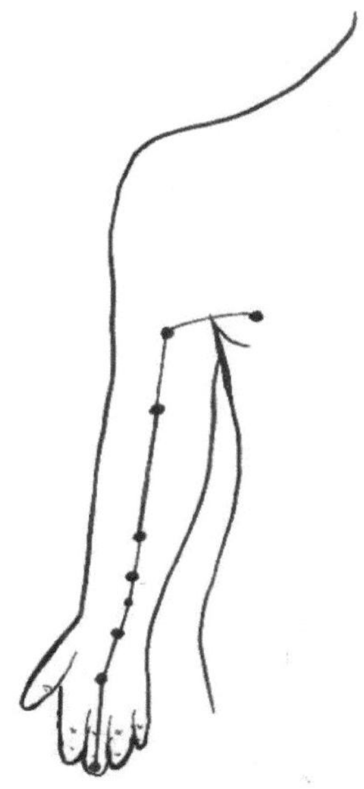

Originates from the chest, the side of the nipple through the armpit and down the arm to the tip of the middle finger. It contains 9 different acupoints.

P-1 (Tianchi 天池)

Indications

Angina pectoris, dysphoria, pain in the hypochondriac region, stomachache, vomiting.

Location

On the chest, in the fourth intercostal space, 1 cun lateral to the nippe, and 5 cun lateral to the anterior midline.

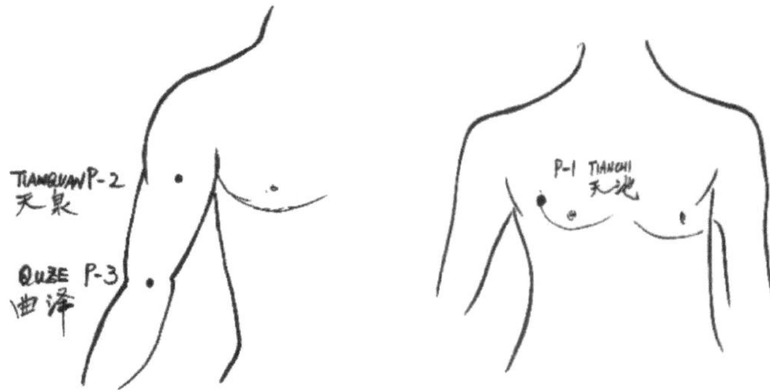

P-2 (Tianquan 天泉)

Indications

Distension of the hypochondriac region, cough, pain in the chest, cardiac pain, back and the medial aspect of the arm.

Location

On the medial side of the arm, 2 cun below the axillary fold, between the two heads of biceps brachii.

P-3 (Quze 曲泽)

- **He-Sea point of the Pericardium channel.**

Indications

Angina pectoris, palpitation, stomachache, vomiting, spasmodic pain of the elbow and forearm.

Location

At the midpoint of the transverse cubital crease, at the ulnar side of the tendon of biceps brachii.

P-4 (Ximen 郄门)

Indications

Angina pectoris, palpitation, hemoptysis, chest pain, epistaxis, epilepsy.

Location

On the palmar side of the forearm, 5 cun above the transverse crease of the wrist, on the line connecting P-3 (Quze 曲泽) and P-7 (Daling 大陵), between the tendons of palmaris longus and flexor carpi radialis.

P-5 (Jianshi 间使)

Indications

Angina pectoris, palpitation, stomachache, vomiting, mania, malaria, epilepsy, contraction of arm and elbow.

Location

On the palmar side of the forearm, 3 cun above the transverse crease of the wrist, on the line connecting P-3 (Quze 曲泽) and P-7 (Daling 大陵), between the tendons of palmaris longus and flexor carpi radialis.

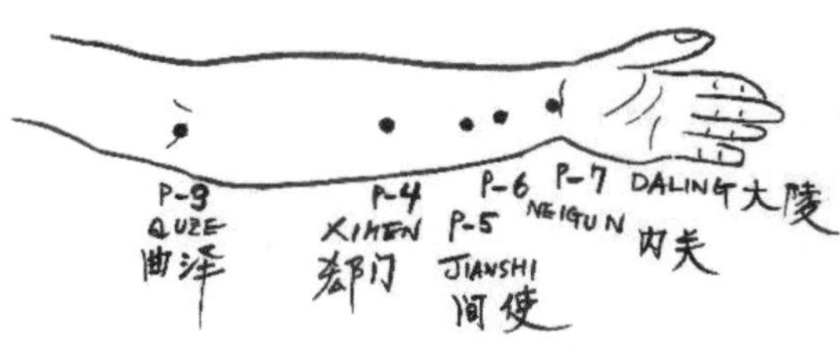

P-6 (Neiguan 内关)

- **Luo-Connecting point of the Pericardium channel.**

Indications

Angina pectoris, palpitation, stomachache, vomiting, nausea, epilepsy, insomnia, mental disorders, spasmodic pain elbow and arm, migraine, febrile disease.

Location

On the palmar side of the forearm, 2 cun above the transverse crease of the wrist, on the line connecting P-3 (Quze 曲泽) and P-7 (Daling 大陵), between the tendons of palmaris longus and flexor carpi radialis.

P-7 (Daling 大陵)

- **Yuan-Source of the Pericardium channel.**

Indications

Angina pectoris, palpitation, stomachache, mania, insomnia, pain in the hypochondriac region, vomiting.

Location

On the palmar side of the forearm, at the midpoint of the transverse crease of the wrist, between the tendons of palmaris longus and flexor carpi radialis.

P-8 (Laogong 劳宫)

Indications

Angina pectoris, palpitation, vomiting, epilepsy, mania, coma due to apoplexy.

Location

On the palm, between the second and third metacarpal bones. When the fist is made, the point is below the tip of the middle finger.

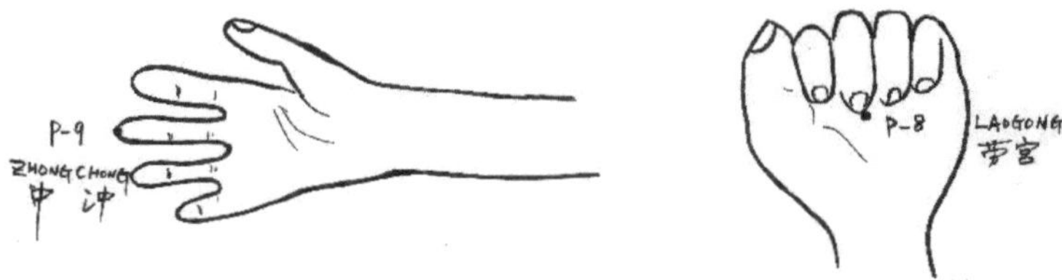

P-9 (Zhongchong 中冲)

- **Jing-Well point**

Indications

Angina pectoris, palpitation, apoplexy, sunstroke, stiffness and swelling of the tongue, febrile disease.

Location

At the center of the tip of the middle finger.

X. The Sanjiao Channel of Hand-Shaoyang
手少阳三焦经经穴

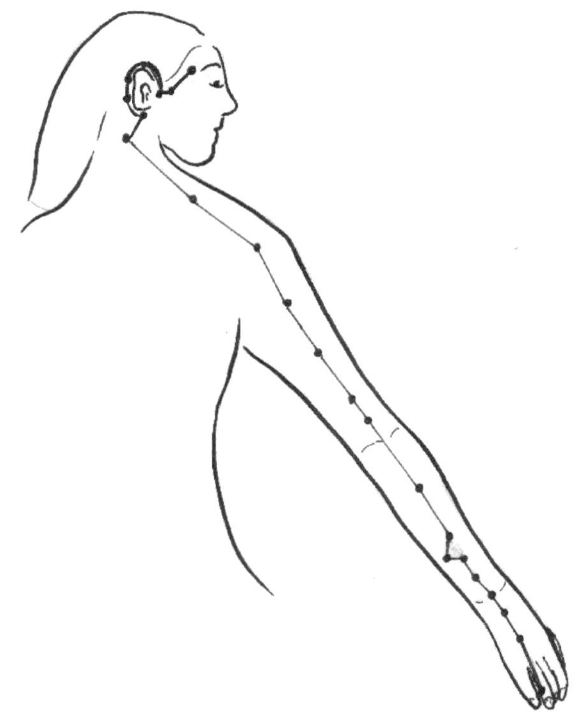

Originates from the tip of the ring finger, runs upward the dorsal aspect of the forearm to the shoulder region and ascends to the neck to the ear, then across the forehead, downward to the cheek to the end of the eyebrow. It contains 23 different acupoints.

SJ-1 (Guanchong 关冲)

- **Jing-Well point**

Indications

Apoplexy, headache, tinnitus, deafness, redness of the eyes.

Location

On the ulnar side of the ring finger, 0.1 cun beside the corner of the nail.

SJ-2 (Yemen 液门)

Indications

Headache, redness of the eyes, tinnitus, deafness, sore throat, numbness of fingers.

Location

When the fist is clenched, between the ring and little fingers, proximal to the margin of the web.

SJ-3 (Zhongzhu 中诸)

Indications

Headache, dizziness, tinnitus, deafness redness of the eyes, sore throat, pain in the elbow and arm, spasmodic pain of the fingers.

Location

On the dorsum of the hand between the fourth and fifth the metacarpal bones, in the depression proximal to the metacarpophalangeal joint, 1 cun posterior to SJ-2 (Yemen 液门).

SJ-4 (Yangchi 阳池)

- **Yuan-Source point of the Sanjiao channel.**

Indications

Tinnitus, deafness, sore throat, pain in the arm, and wrist, flaccidity and Bi syndrome of the upper limbs, diabetes.

Location

On the dorsum of the wrist, in the depression between the tendons of extensor digitorum communis and extensor digiti minimi.

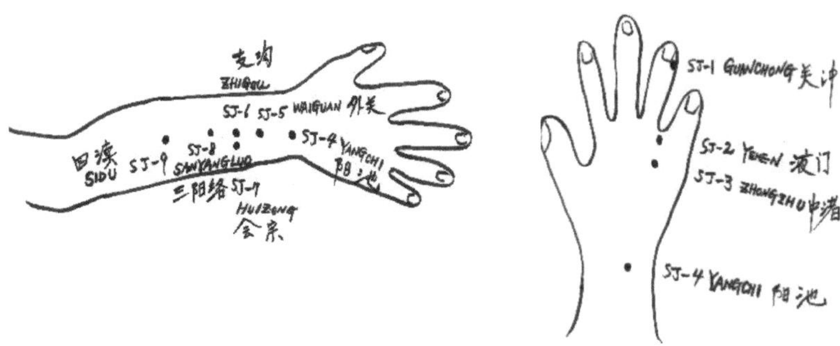

SJ-5 (Waiguan 外关)

- **Luo-Connecting point of the Sanjiao channel.**

Indications

Deafness, tinnitus, migraine, pain in the cheek, headache, febrile disease, motor impairment of the elbow and arm.

Location

On the dorsum of the forearm, on the line connecting SJ-4 (Yangchi 阳池) and olecranon, 2 cun proximal to the dorsal crease of the wrist, between the radius and the ulna.

SJ-6 (Zhigou 支沟)

Indications

Tinnitus, deafness, pain in the shoulder and back, sudden loss of voice, pain in the hypochondriac region, constipation, vomiting.

Location

On the dorsum of the forearm, on the line connecting SJ-4 (Yangchi 阳池) and olecranon, 3 cun proximal to the dorsal crease of the wrist, between the radius and the ulna.

SJ-7 (Huizong 会宗)

- **Xi-Cleft point of the Sanjiao channel.**

Indications

Pain in the ear, deafness, pain in the upper limbs.

Location

On the dorsum of the forearm, at the same level with SJ-6 (Zhigou 支沟), on the radial border of the ulna.

SJ-8 (Sanyangluo 三阳络)

Indications

Deafness, sudden loss of voice, pain in the upper limbs.

Location

On the dorsum of the forearm, 4 cun above the transverse crease, between the ulna and the radius.

SJ-9 (Sidu 四读)

Indications

Deafness, sudden loss of voice, pain in the upper limbs.

Location

On the dorsum of the forearm, 7 cun proximal to SJ-4 (Yangchi 阳池), in the depression between the radius and the ulna.

SJ-10 (Tianjing 天井)

- **He-Sea point of the sanjiao channel.**

Indications

Migraine, pain in the shoulder and arm, epilepsy, hypochondriac pain.

Location

With the elbow flexed, in the depression 1 cun proximal to the tip of the olecranon.

SJ-11 (Qinglengyuan 请冷渊)

Indications

Migraine, pain in the shoulder and arm.

Location

With the elbow flexed, 1 cun proximal to SJ-10 (Tianjing 天井).

SJ-12 (Xiaoluo 消泺)

Indications

Headache, motor impairment of the arm. Neck rigidity.

Location

On the upper arm, on the line connecting SJ-10 (Tianjing 天井) and SJ-14 (Jianliao 肩髎), 4 cun proximal to SJ-10 (Tianjing 天井).

SJ-13 (Naohui 臑会)

Indications

Pain in the shoulder and arm, goiter.

Location

On the lateral side of the upper arm, on the line connecting the tip of the olecranon and SJ-14 (Jianliao 肩髎), 3 cun below SJ-14 (Jianliao 肩髎).

SJ-14 (Jianliao 肩髎)

Indications

Pain and motor impairment of the shoulder and arm.

Location

On the posterior side of the shoulder, posterior to SJ-14 (Jianliao 肩髎), the point is in the depression inferior and posterior to the acromion when the arm is abducted.

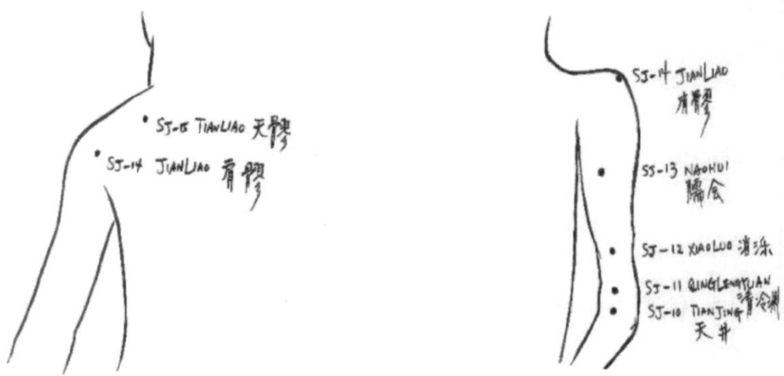

SJ-15 (Tianliao 天髎)

Indications

Pain in the shoulder and elbow, stiffness of the neck.

Location

On the scapula, midway between GB-21 (Jianjing 肩井) and SI-13 (Quyuan 曲垣), 1 cun below GB-21 (Jianjing 肩井).

SJ-16 (Tianyou 天牖)

Indications

Headache, neck, rigidity, blurred vision, sudden deafness.

Location

On the lateral side of the neck, directly below the posterior border of the mastoid process. On the level of the mandibular angle, on the posterior border of the sternocleidomastoid muscle, 1 cun inferior to GB-12 (Wangu 完骨).

SJ-17 (Yifeng 翳风)

Indications

Tinnitus, deafness, facial paralysis, toothache, hiccup.

Location

Behind the earlobe, in the depression between the mandible and mastoid process.

SJ-18 (Chimai 瘛脉)

Indications

Headache, tinnitus, deafness.

Location

On the head, in the depression on the mastoid bone, at the junction of the middle third and lower third of the distance, along the curve of the ear helix from SJ-17 (Yifeng 翳风) to SJ-20 (Jiaosun 角孙), and divide this curved line into three equal parts, and form four points.

SJ-19 (Luxi 颅息)

Indications

Headache, tinnitus, deafness, pain in the ear.

Location

On the head, at the junction of the upper and middle third of the curv formed by SJ-17 (Yifeng 翳风) and SJ-20 (Jiaosun 角孙) behind the felix.

SJ-20 (Jiaosun 角孙)

Indications

Migraine, tinnitus, deafness, cataract, toothache, swelling of cheeks.

Location

Directly above the ear apex, within the hair line.

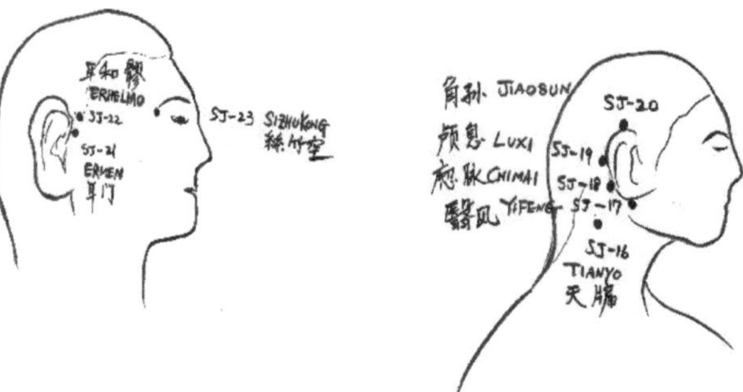

SJ-21 (Ermen 耳门)

Indications

Tinnitus, deafness, toothache, otorrhea, swelling of the cheeks.

Location

On the face, anterior to the supratragic notch, with the mouth open, the point is in the depression superior to the condyloid process of the mandible.

SJ-22 (Erheliao 耳和髎)

Indications

Migraine, tinnitus, deafness.

Locations

On the lateral side of the head, the point is the intersection of the level line from the upper border of the root of ear forward and the posterior border of the hairline of the temple.

SJ-23 (Sizhukong 丝竹空)

Indications

Headache, dizziness, toothache, blurred vision, epilepse, swelling pain of the eyes.

Location

In the depression at the lateral end of the eyebrow.

XI. The Gallbladder Channel of Foot-Shaoyang 足少阳胆经经

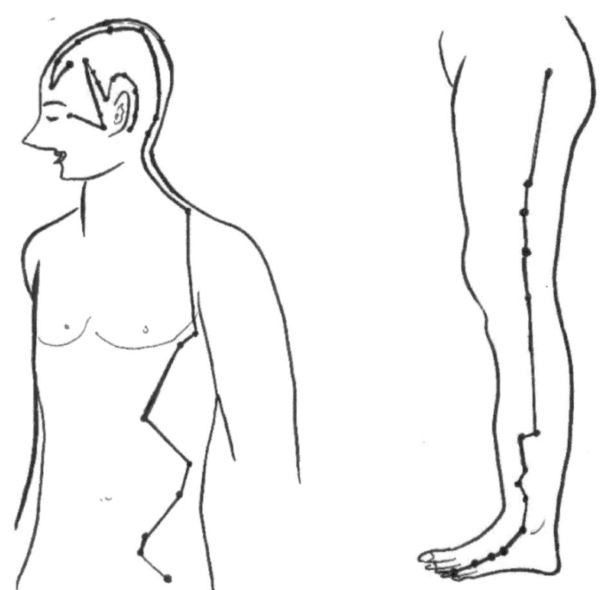

Originates from outer canthus, ascends to the corner of the forehead, back and forth across the skull and then runs down the neck across the shoulder and zigzags back and forth across the chest and abdomen. From there it descends along the lateral aspect of the thigh to the knee, and reaches the anterior aspect of the externa malleolus, and then follow to the tip of the fourth toe. It contains 44 different acupoints.

GB-1 (Tongziliao 瞳子髎)

Indications

> Headache, pain and swelling of eyes, cataract, glaucoma, headache, epiphora.

122

Location

0.5 cun lateral to the outer canthus, in the depression lateral to the orbit.

GB-2 (Tinghui 听会)

Indications

Tinnitus, deafness, toothache, headache, swelling and pain the cheeks.

Location

On the face, anterior to the intertragic notch. When the mouth is opened, the point is located in a depression appeared.

GB-3 (Shangguan 上关)

Indications

Tinnitus, deafness, toothache, migraine, toothache, deviation of the mouth and eye.

Location

Anterior to the ear, in a depression above the upper border of the zygomatic arch.

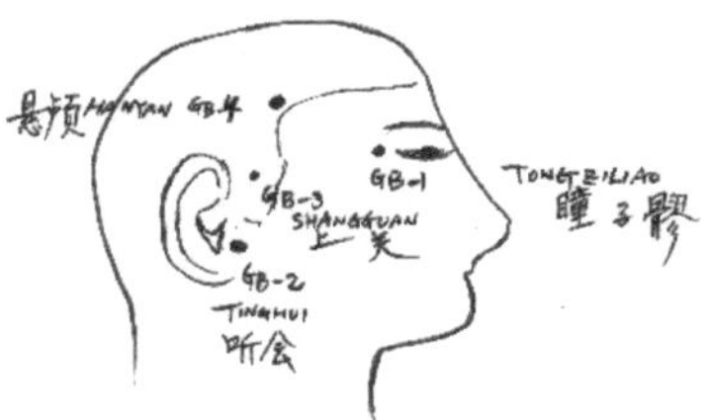

GB-4 (Hanyan 頷厌)

Indications

Migraine, tinnitus, vertigo, epilepsy, toothache, pain in the outer canthus.

Location

In the temporal region, within the hairline, at the junction of the upper ¼ and lower ¾ of the curved line linking ST-8 (Touwei 头维) and GB-7 (Qubin 曲鬓).

GB-5 (Xuanlu 悬颅)

Indications

Migraine, redness, swelling and pain of eyes, toothache.

Location

In the temporal region, within the hairline, at the midpoint of the curved line connecting ST-8 (Touwei 头维) and GB-7 (Qubin 曲鬓).

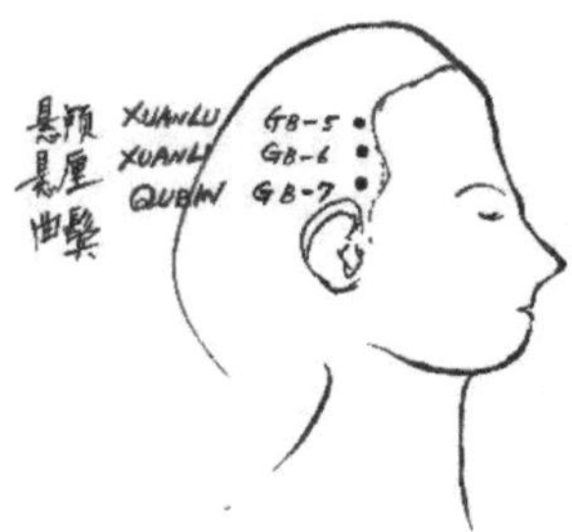

GB-6 (Xuanli 悬厘)

Indications

Migraine, tinnitus, pain in the outer canthus.

Location

In the temporal region, within the hairline, at the junction of the upper ¾ and lower ¼ of the curved line connecting ST-8 (Touwei 头维) and GB-7 (Qubin 曲鬓).

GB-7 (Qubin 曲鬓)

Indications

Migraine, toothache, swelling of the cheek, headache.

Location

In the temporal region, within the hairline, one index finger-breadth anterior to SJ-20 (Jiaosun 角孙).

GB-8 (Shuaigu 率谷)

Indications

Migraine, vertigo, vomiting, infantile convulsion.

Location

On the head, 1.5 cun superior to the hairline above SJ-20 (Jiaosun 角孙).

GB-9 (Tianchong 天冲)

Indications

Headache, epilepsy, swelling and pain of the gums, convulsion.

Location

Directly above the ear, in the depression 0.5 cun posterior to GB-8 (Shuaigu 率谷).

GB-10 (Fubai 浮白)

Indications

Headache, tinnitus, deafness.

Location

Posterior and superior to the mastoid process, draw a curved line along the auricle from GB-9 (Tianchong 天冲) to GB-12 (Wangu 完骨), at the junction of the middle third and upper third of the curve line.

GB-11 (Touqiaoyin 头窍阴)

Indications

Tinnitus, deafness, pain in the ears, head and neck.

Location

Posterior and superior to the mastoid process, at the junction of middle one-third and lower one-third of the curved line connecting GB-9 (Tianchong 天冲) and GB-12 (Wangu 完骨).

GB-12 (Wangu 完骨)

Indications

Headache, stiffness and pain of neck, epilepsy, malaria, toothache, insomnia, deviation of the eye and mouth.

Location

In the depression posterior and inferior to the mastoid process.

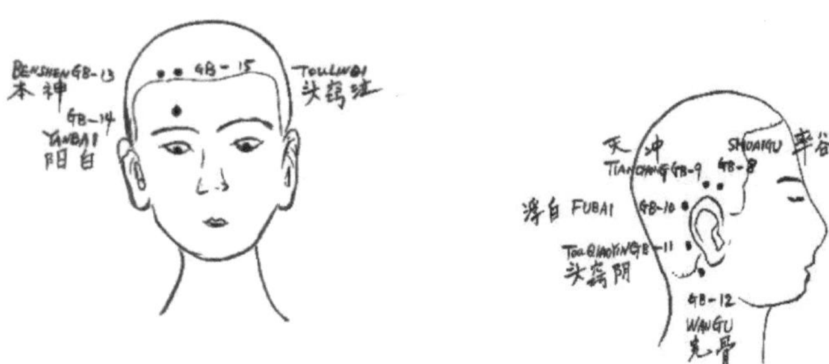

GB-13 (Benshen 本神)

Indications

Headache, insomnia, vertigo, epilepsy.

Location

On the forehead, 0.5 cun within the anterior hairline, 3 cun lateral to DU-24 (Shenting 神庭).

GB-14 (Yangbai 阳白)

Indications

Pain of eyes, blurred vision, headache in frontal region, twitchcingof the eyelids.

Location

On the forehead, directly above the pupil, 1 cun superior to the middle of the eyebrow.

GB-15 (Toulinqi 头临泣)

Indications

Headache, vertigo, rhinorrhea, pain in the outer canthus, nasal obstruction, cataract, tinnitus, deafness, infantile convulsion.

Location

On the forehead, directly above GB-14 (Yangbai 阳白), 0.5 cun within the anterior hairline.

GB-16 (Muchuang 目窗)

Indications

Headache, vertigo, red and painful eyes, nasal obstruction.

Location

1.5 cun within the anterior hairline, 2.25 cun lateral to the midline of the head.

GB-17 (Zhengying 正营)

Indications

Migraine, vertigo.

Location

2.5 cun within the anterior hairline, 2.25 cun lateral to the midline of the head.

GB-18 (Chengling 承灵)

Indications

Headache, vertigo, epilepsy, rhinorrhea.

Location

4 cun within the anterior hairline, 2.25 cun lateral to the midline of the head.

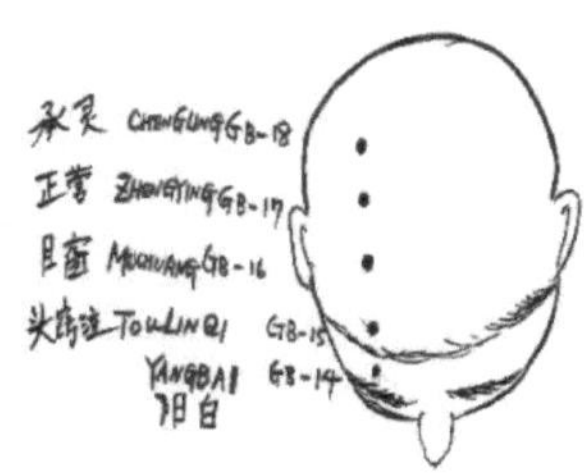

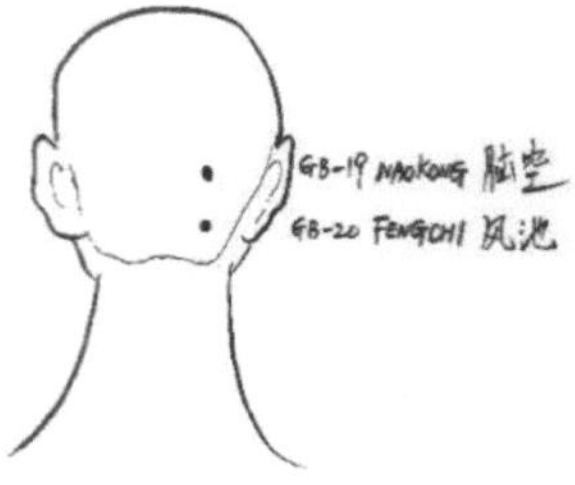

GB-19 (Naokong 脑空)

Indications

Headache, stiffness, of the neck, vertigo, tinnitus, epilepsy, pain of eyes.

Location

On the occipital region, 2.25 cun lateral to the midlineof the head, level as DU-17 (Naohu 脑户).

GB-20 (Fengchi 风池)

Indications

Headache, vertigo, redness, swelling and pain of eyes, rhinorrhea, epistaxis, tinnitus, deafness, glaucoma, epilepsy, febrile diseases, common cold, nasal obstruction.

Location

Below the occiput, at the same level as Du-16 (Fengfu 风府), in the depression between the origins of the sternocleidomastoid and trapezius muscles.

GB-21 (Jianjing 肩井)

Indications

Stiffness and pain of neck, shoulder, paralysis of upper limbs, scrofula, apoplexy.

Location

On the shoulder, directly above the nipple, midway between DU-14(Dazhui 大椎) and the tip of the acromion.

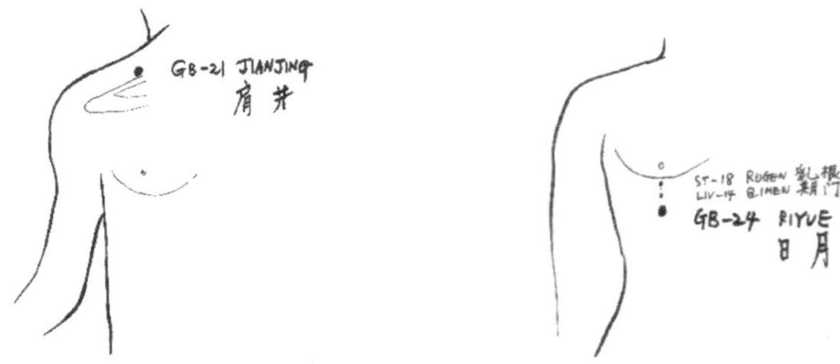

GB-22 (Yuanye 渊腋)

Indications

Pain and paralysis of the arm, fullness of the chest.

Location

On the lateral side of the chest, on the axillary midline when the arm is raised, 3 cun below the axilla, at the level of the nipple, in the 4th intercostal space.

GB-23 (Zhejin 辄筋)

Indications

Pain in the hypochondriac region, fullness of the chest, pain and paralysis of the arm.

Location

1 cun anterior to GB-22 (Yuanye 渊腋), at the level of the nipple, in the 4th intercostal space.

GB-24 (Riyue 日月)

- **Front-Mu point of the Gall Bladder.**

Indications

Jaundice, hypochondriac pain, vomiting, acid regurgitation, hiccup, vomiting.

Location

Directly below the nipple, in the 7th intercostal space, 4 cun lateral to the midline.

GB-25 (Jingmen 京门)

- **Front-Mu point of the Kidney.**

Indications

Abdominal distension, diarrhea, borborygmus, hypochondriac pain, edema, lumbago, dysuria.

Location

On the lower border of the free end of the 12th rib.

GB-26 (Daimai 带脉)

Indications

Amenorrhea, irregular menstruation, leukorrhea, hernia, abdominal pain, pain in the hypochondriac region.

Location

On the lateral side of the abdomen, directly below LIV-13(Zhangmen 章门), at the level of the umbilicus.

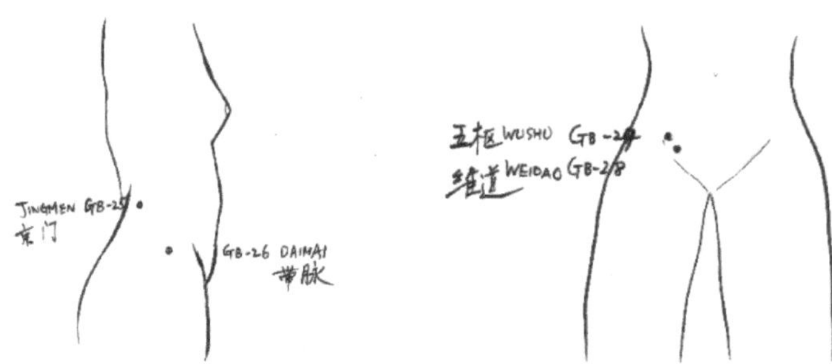

GB-27 (Wushu 五俞)

Indications

Lower abdominal pain, leukorrhea, hernia, constipation.

Location

On the lateral side of the abdomen, anterior to the superior iliac spine, 3 cun below the level of the umbilicus, level with REN-4 (Guanyuan 关元).

GB-28 (Weidao 维道)

Indications

Lower abdominal pain, leukorrhea, hernia.

Location

On the lateral side of the abdomen, 0.5 cun anterior and inferior to GB-27 (Wushu 五俞), on the line parallel to the groin.

GB-29 (Juliao 居髎)

Indications

Hernia, lumbago, muscular atrophy of the lower limbs.

Location

On the hip, at the midpoint of the line connecting the anterior superior iliac spine and the prominence of the greater trochanter.

GB-30 (Huantiao 环跳)

Indications

Pain of the lumbar region and thigh, muscular atrophy of the lower limbs, sprain of waist, urticaria.

Location

On the postero-lateral side of the hip joint, one third of the distance between the prominence of the great trochanter and the sacrococcygeal hiatus.

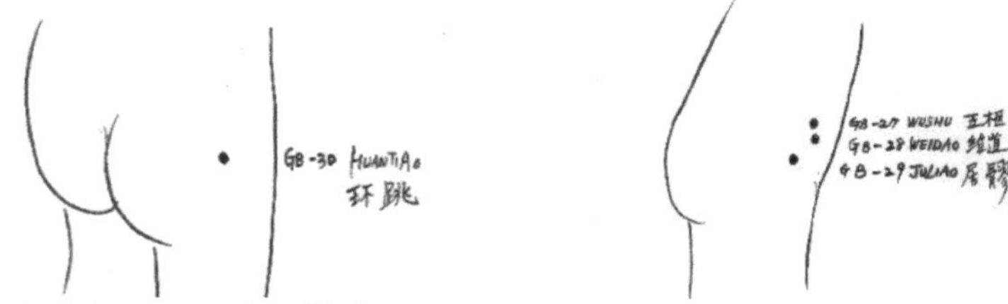

GB-31 (Fengshi 风市)

Indications

Paralysis of the lower limbs, beriberi, general pruritus, beriberi.

Location

On the lateral midline of the thigh, 7 cun superior to the popliteal crease, when the patient stands erect with the arms hanging down freely, the point is the tip of the middle finger.

GB-32 (Zhongdu 中读)

Indications

Hemiplegia, numbness and weakness of the lower limbs, pain and soreness of the thigh and knee.

Location

On the lateral side of the thigh, 2 cun inferior to GB-31 (Fengshi 风市).

GB-33 (Xiyangguan 膝阳关)

Indications

Swelling and pain of the knee, numbness of the leg.

Location

On the lateral side of the knee, 3 cun above GB-34 (Yanglingquan 阳陵泉), at the level of the upper border of the patella, in the depression above the external epicondyle of femur.

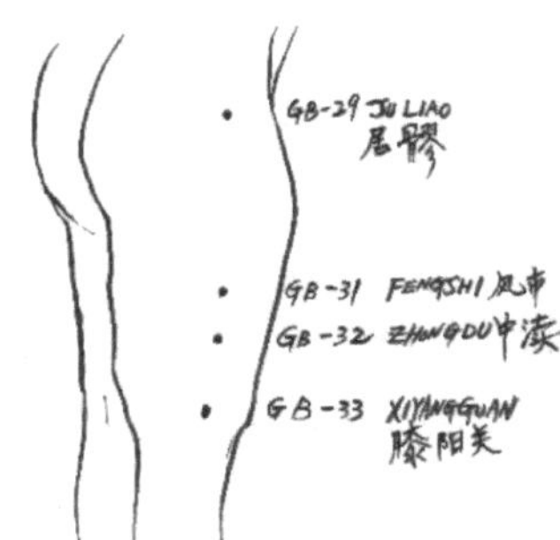

GB-34 (Yanglingquan 阳陵泉)

- **He-Sea point of the Gall Bladder channel.**

Indications

Hypochondriac pain, bitter taste in the mouth, jaundice, vomiting, hemiplegia, swelling and pain of the knee, numbness of the lower extremities.

Location

On the lateral side of the lower leg, in the depression anterior and inferior to the head of the fibula.

GB-35 (Yangjiao 阳交)

Indications

Distension and fullness in the chest and hypochondria, muscular atrophy and paralysis of the leg, mania, depression.

Location

On the lateral side of the lower leg, 7 cun above to the prominence of the lateral malleolus, on the posterior border of the fibula.

GB-36 (Waiqiu 外丘)

- **Xi-Cleft point of the Gall Bladder channel.**

Indications

Fullness and distension in the chest, pain in the hypochondriac region, mania, despression.

Location

On the lateral aspect of the lower leg, 7 cun superior to the prominence of the lateral malleolus, on the anterior border of the fibula.

GB-37 (Guangming 光明)

- **Luo-connecting point of the Gall Bladder channel.**

Indications

Blurred vision, pain of eyes, night blindness, distending pain in the breast, muscular atrophy, motor impairment and pain of the lower extremities.

Location

On the lateral side of the lower leg, 5 cun superior to the prominence of the lateral malleolus, on the anterior border of the fibula.

GB-38 (Yangfu 阳辅)

Indicaations

Migraine, pain of the outer canthus, pain in the axillary region, distending pain in the chest and hypochondriac region.

Location

On the lateral side of the lower leg, 4 cun superior to the prominence of the lateral malleolus, on the anterior border of the fibula.

GB-39 (Xuanzhong 悬钟)

Indications

Stiffness of neck, pain in the chest and hypochondria, sore throat, beriberi, hemorrhoids, muscular atrophy of the lower limbs.

Location

On the lateral side of the lower leg, 3 cun superior to the prominence of the lateral malleolus, on the anterior border of the fibula.

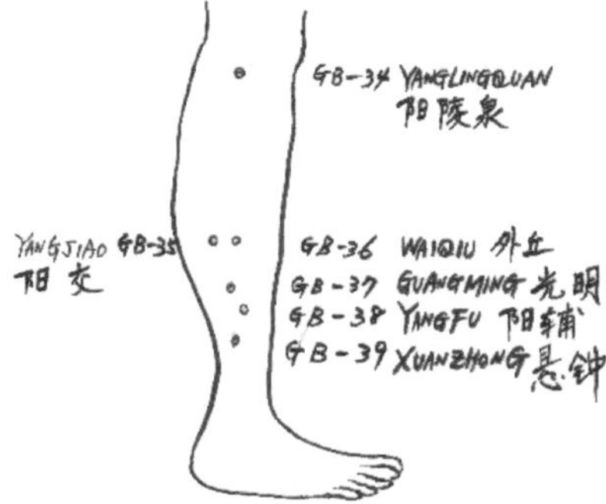

GB-40 (Qiuxu 丘墟)

- **Yuan-Source point of the Gall Bladder channel.**

Indications

Pain in the hypochondriac region, vomiting acid regurgitation, muscular atrophy of the lower limbs, malaria, swelling and pain of the external malleolus.

Location

At the ankle joint, anterior and inferior to the lateral malleolus.

GB-41 (Zulinqi 足临泣)

Indications

Hypochondriac pain, numbness of toes, pain of foot dorsum, numbness of toes, irregular menstruation, pain and swelling of eyes.

Location

On the lateral side of the dorsum of the foot, 4th and 5th metatarsal bones, in a depression lateral to the tendon of the extensor digitiform longus of the fifth toe.

GB-42 (Diwuhui 地五会)

Indications

Pain of the canthus, tinnitus, swelling and pain of foot dorsum, distending pain of the breast.

Location

Between the 4th and 5th metatarsal bones, on the medial side of the tendon of extensor digitorum longus.

GB-43 (Xiaxi 侠溪)

Indications

Headache, vertigo, tinnitus, deafness, swelling and pain of the eyes, pain in the hypochondria, distending pain of the breast, febrile diseases.

Location

Between the fourth and fifth toes, 0.5 cun proximal to the margin of the web.

GB-44 (Zuqiaoyin 足窍阴)

- **Jing-Well point**

Indications

Headache, redness, swelling and pain of eyes, migraine, deafness, tinnitus, febrile diseases, insomnia, hypochondriac pain apoplexy, sore throat.

Location

On the lateral side of the fourth toe, 0.1 cun from the corner of the nail.

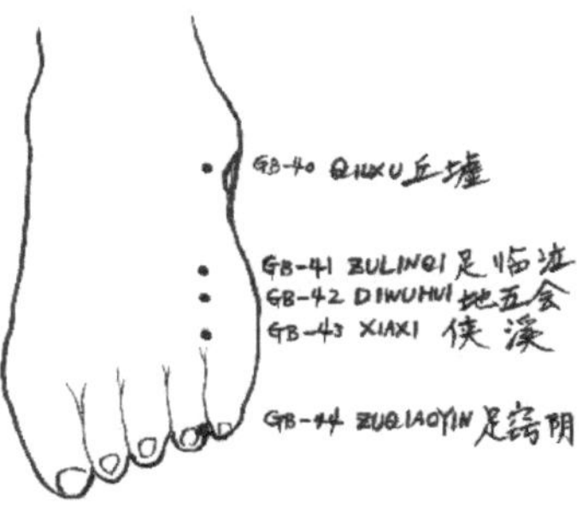

XII. The Liver Channel of Foot-Jueyin 足厥阴肝经经穴

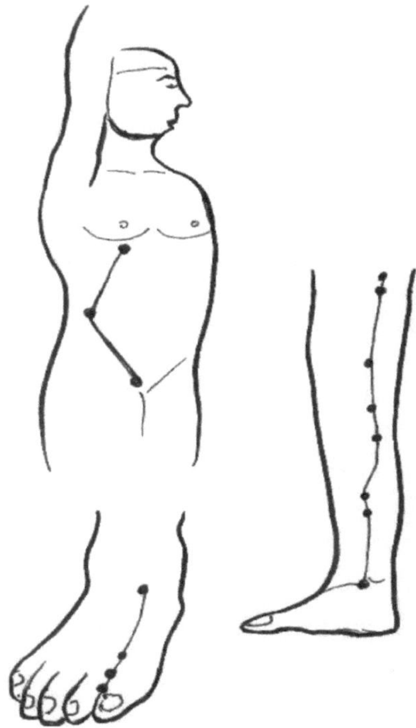

Originates from the dorsal region of the great toe, and then runs upward along the foot, leg to the groin and then runs upward around the stomach up to just below the nipple. It contains 14 different acupoints.

LIV-1 (Dadun 大敦)

- **Jing-Well point**

Indications

Apoplexy, epilepsy, hernia, coma, irregular menstruation, metrorrhagia, metrostaxis, contraction of genitalia.

Location

On the lateral side of dorsum of the the great toe, 0.1 cun beside the corner of the nail.

LIV-2 (Xingjian 行间)

Indications

Abdominal distension, headache, vertigo, redness and swelling pain of eyes, glaucoma, hernia, jaundice, irregular menstruation, metrorrhagia, metrostaxis, epilepsy, insomnia, pain and swelling in the dorsum of foot, numbness of toes.

Location

On the lateral side of dorsum of the foot, between the first and second toes, 0.5 cun proximal of the margin of the web.

LIV-3 (Taichong 太冲)

- **Yuan-Source of the Liver channel.**

Indications

Headache, vertigo, dizziness, pain and swelling of the eyes, glaucoma, nearsightedness, facial paralysis, hernia, vomiting, pain in the hypochondriac region, epilepsy, apoplexy, flaccidity of lower limbs, severe lumbago, infantile convulsion.

Location

On the dorsum of the foot, in the depression distal to the junction, between the first and second metatarsal bones.

LIV-4 (Zhongfeng 中封)

Indications

Hernia, retention of urine, metrorrhagia, metrostaxis, irregular menstruation, jaundice.

Location

On the ankle, anterior to the medial malleolus, in the depression on the medial side of the tendon of the m.tibialis anterior.

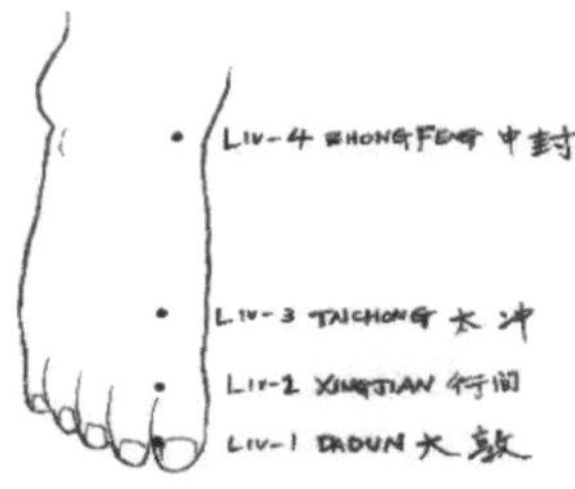

LIV-5 (Ligou 蠡溝)

- **Luo-Connecting point of the Liver channel.**

Indications

Irregular menstruation, leukorrhea, pruritus valvae, unsmooth urination, hernia, lower abdominal pain.

Location

5 cun above the prominence of the medial malleolus, in the middle of the medial aspect of the tibia.

LIV-6 (Zhongdu 中都)

- **Xi-Cleft point of the Liver channel.**

Indications

Abdominal pain, hypochondriac pain, diarrhea, hernia, metrorrhagia, metrostaxis.

Location

7 cun above the prominence of the medial malleolus, on the midline of the medial aspect of the tibia.

LIV-7 (Xiguan 膝关)

Indication

Pain and swelling of the knee.

Location

Posterior and inferior to the medial epicondyle of the tibia, 1 cun posterior to SP-9 (Yinlingquan 阴陵泉).

LIV-8 (Ququan 曲泉)

- **He-Sea point of the Liver channel.**

Indications

Irregular menstruation, dysmenorrhea, leukorrhea, pruritus vulvae, pain and swelling of the knee.

Location

When the knee is flexed, in the depression above the medial end of the transverse crease of the knee joint.

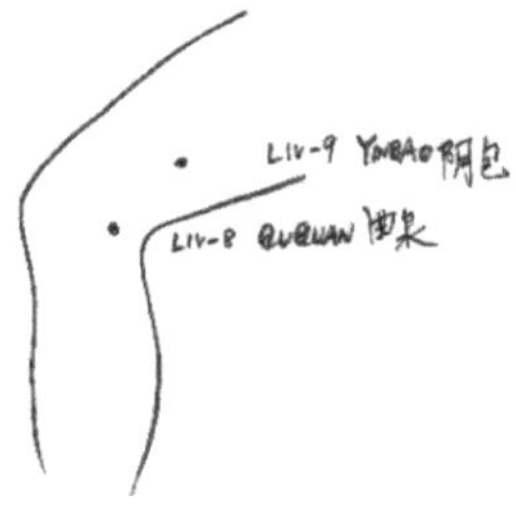

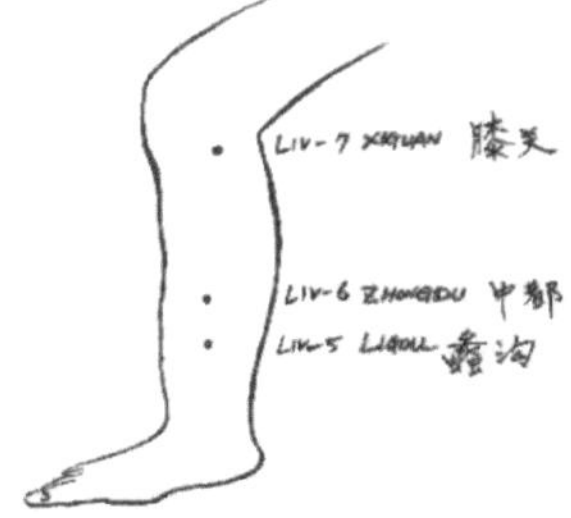

LIV-9 (Yinbao 阴包)

Indications

Lower abdominal pain, enuresis, pain in the lumbosacral region, irregular menstruation, retention of urine.

Location

On the medial side of the thigh, directly above the medial epicondyle of the femur, 4 cun above to LIV-8 (Ququan 曲泉).

LIV-10 (Zuwuli 足五里)

Indications

Lower abdominal distension, retention of urine.

Location

3 cun directly below ST-30 (Qichong 气冲), at the proximal end of the thigh, below the pubic tubercle and on the lateral border of m.adductor longus.

LIV-11 (Yinlian 阴廉)

Indications

Irregular menstruation, leukorrhea, lower abdominal pain, pain in the thigh and leg.

Location

2 cun directly below ST-30 (Qichong 气冲), at the proximal end of the thigh, below the pubic tubercle and on the lateral border of m.adductor longus.

LIV-12 (Jimai 急脉)

Indications

Lower abdominal pain, hernia, pain in the external genitalia.

Location

2.5 cun lateral to the midway of the lower border of the pubic symphysis, 1 cun inferior to Ren-2 (Qugu 曲骨).

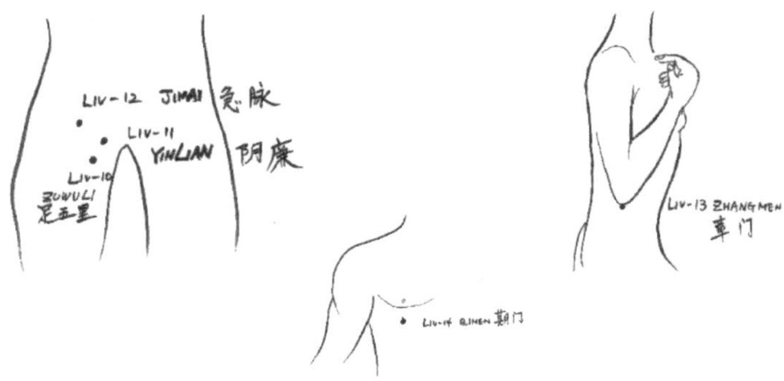

LIV-13 (Zhangmen 章门)

Indications

Abdominal pain and distension, borborygmus, diarrhea, vomiting, hypochondriac pain.

Location

On the lateral side of the abdomen, when the patient is flexing elbow, and touching the tip of the elbow to the hypochondriac region, the tip of the elbow.

LIV-14 (Qimen 期门)

- **Front-Mu point of the Liver.**

Indications

Hypochondriac pain, abdominal distension, vomiting, hiccup, acid regurgitation, breast abscess, depression.

Location

Directly below the nipple, in the 6th intercostal space, 4 cun lateral to the midline.

XIII.Point of the Du Channel 督脉经穴

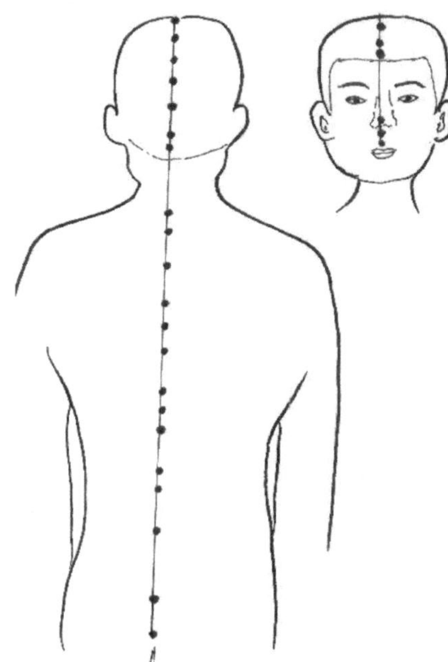

Originates from the lower abdomen and emerges from the perineum and runs straight up the spinal column to the nape, over the skull to above lip. It contains 28 different acupoints.

DU-1 (Changqiang 长强)

- **Luo-Connecting point of the Governing vessel.**

Indications

Constipation, hemorrhoids, prolapse of rectum, diarrhea, hematochezia, mania, depression, epilepsy, pain in the lower back.

Location

At the midpoint between the tip of the coccyx and the anus.

DU-2 (Yaoshu 腰俞)

Indications

Stiffness and pain of the lower back, irregular menstruation, hemorrhoids, epilepsy, muscular atrophy of the lower extremities.

Location

On the sacrum, on the midline, at the sacral hiatus.

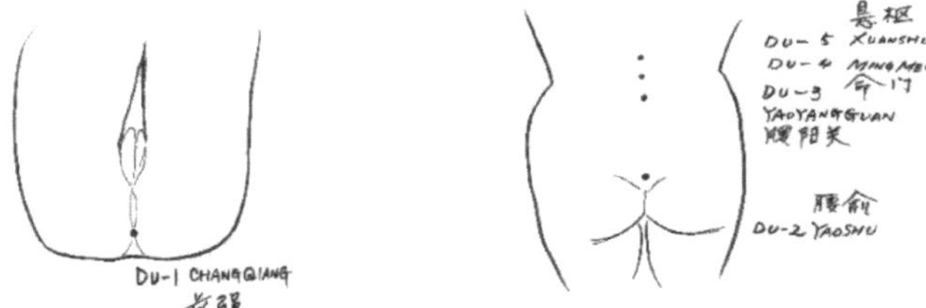

DU-3 (Yaoyangguan 腰阳关)

Indications

Irregular menstruation, impotence, seminal emission, muscular atrophy of the lower extremities.

Location

On the lower back, in the depression below the spinous process of the fourth lumbar vertebra.

DU-4 (Mingmen 命门)

Indications

Stiffness of the back, lumbago, leukorrhea, impotence, seminal emission, diarrhea.

Location

On the lower back, in the depression below the spinous process of the second lumbar vertebra.

DU-5 (Xuanshu 悬俞)

Indications

Pain and stiffness of the lower back, diarrhea, indigestion.

Location

On the lower back, in the depression below the spinous process of the first lumbar vertebra.

DU-6 (Jizhong 脊中)

Indications

Epilepsy, diarrhea, jaundice, hemorrhoids, stiffness and pain of the back, pain in the epigastric region.

Location

On the back, in the depression below the spinous process of the eleventh thoracic vertebra.

DU-7 (Zhongshu 中俞)

Indications

Pain in the epigastric region, low back pain, stiffness of the back.

Location

On the back, in the depression below the spinous process of the tenth thoracic vertebra.

DU-8 (Jinsuo 筋缩)

Indications

Stomachache, jaundice, stiffness of the back, depression, mania.

Location

On the back, in the depression below the spinous process of the ninth thoracic vertebra.

DU-9 (Zhiyang 至阳)

Indications

Pain in the chest and back, jaundice, cough, asthma.

Location

On the back, in the depression below the spinous process of the seventh thoracic vertebra.

DU10 (Lingtai 灵台)

Indications

Cough, asthma, stiffness of the back and carbuncle.

Location

On the back, in the depression below the spinous process of the sixth thoracic vertebra.

DU-11 (Shendao 神道)

Indications

Stiffness and pain in the back, cough, asthma, angina pectoris, palpitation, insomnia.

Location

On the back, in the depression below the spinous process of the fifth thoracic vertebra.

DU-12 (Shenzhu 身柱)

Indications

Cough, asthma, epilepsy, stiffness and pain in the back.

Location

On the back, in the depression below the spinous process of the third thoracic vertebra.

DU-13 (Taodao 陶道)

Indications

Cough, asthma, epilepsy, mania, febrile diseases, headache, malaria, backcarbuncle.

Location

On the back, in the depression below the spinous process of the first thoracic vertebra.

DU-14 (Dazhui 大椎)

- **Point of the Sea of Qi.**
- **Meeting point of the Governing vessel with Six Yang channel.**

Indications

Malaria, febrile diseases, common cold, afternoon fever, cough, asthma, epilepsy, stiffness of the neck.

Location

At the level of the shoulder, in the depression below the spinous process of the seventh cervical vertebra.

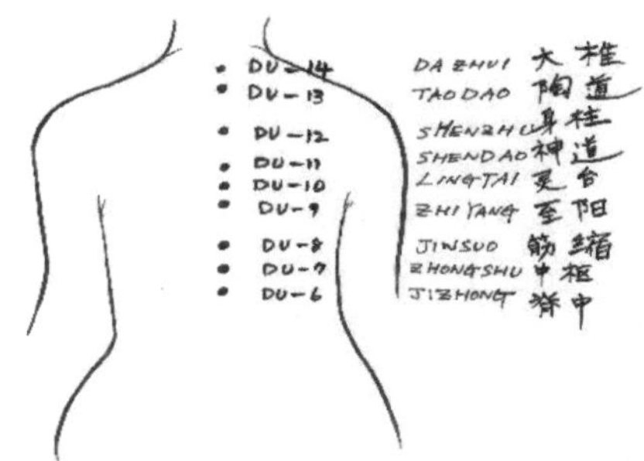

DU-15 (Yamen 哑门)

Indications

Epilepsy, mental disorder, headache, stiff neck, sudden loss of voice, stiffness of the tongue and aphasia due to apoplexy.

Location

On the neck, 0.5 cun above the midpoint of the posterior hairline, below the first cervical vertebra.

DU-16 (Fengfu 风府)

- **Point of the Sea of Marrow.**

Indications

Epilepsy, headache, dizziness, stiff neck, hemiplegia, inability to speak after apoplexy, sore throat.

Location

On the neck, 1cun above the midpoint of the posterior hairline, below the external occipital protuberance.

DU-17 (Naohu 脑户)

Indications

Headache, dizziness, loss of voice, mania, depression, stiffness of the neck.

Location

On the head, 2.5 cun above the midpoint of the posterior hairline, 1.5 cun above DU-16 (Fengfu 风府), in the depression superior to the external occipital protuberance.

DU-18 (Qiangjian 强间)

Indications

Headache, vertigo, epilepsy, stiff neck, insomnia, mania.

Location

On the head, 4 cun above the midpoint of the posterior hairline, 1.5 cun above DU-17 (Naohu 脑户).

DU-19 (Houding 后顶)

Indications

Headache, vertigo, stiffness of the neck, epilepsy, depression, mania.

Location

On the head, 5.5 cun above the midpoint of the posterior hairline, 1.5 cun above DU-18 (Qiangjian 强间).

DU-20 (Baihui 白会)

- **Point of the Sea of Marrow.**

Indications

Headache, vertigo, wind stroke, mental disorders, Insomnia, prolapse of rectum, nasal obstruction, tinnitus.

Location

On the midline of the head, 5 cun above the midpoint of the anterior hairline, at the midpoint connecting the apexes of both ears.

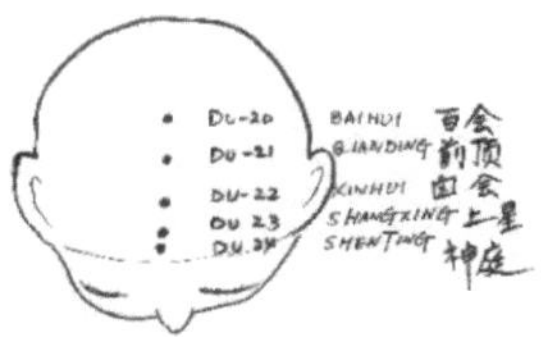

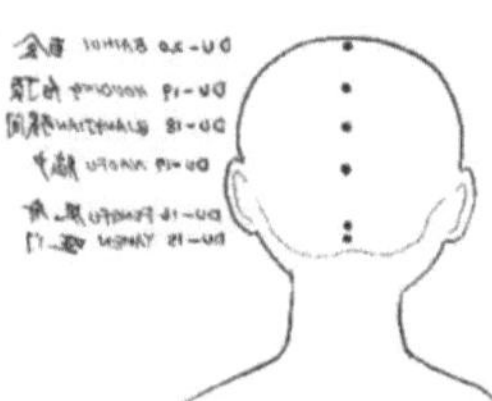

DU-21 (Qianding 前顶)

Indications

Headache, vertigo, rhinorrhea, blurred vision, epilepsy.

Location

On the head, 3.5 cun above the midpoint of the anterior hairline, 1.5 cun anterior to DU-20 (Baihui 白会).

DU-22 (Xinhui 囟会)

Indications

Headache, blurred vision, rhinorrhea, epistaxis.

Location

On the head, 2 cun above the midpoint of the anterior hairline, 3 cun anterior to DU-20 (Baihui 白会).

DU-23 (Shangxing 上星)

Indications

Headache, vertigo, rhinorrhea, epilepsy, epistaxis, pain of eyes.

Location

On the head, 1 cun above the midpoint of the anterior hairline.

DU-24 (Shenting 神庭)

Indications

Headache, vertigo, insomnia, epistaxis, cataract, palpitation, insomnia, rhinorrhea, mental disorders.

Location

At the top of the head, 0.5 cun above the midpoint of the anterior hairline.

DU-25 (Suliao 素髎)

Indications

Loss of consciousness, rhinorrhea, epistaxis, nasal obstruction.

Location

On the face, on the tip of the nose.

DU-26 (Shuigou 水沟)

Indications

Epilepsy, apoplexy, unconsciousness, mental disorders, infantile convulsion, nasal obstruction, stiff neck, infantile enuresis.

Location

Above the upper lip on the midline, at the junction of the upper third and middle third of the philtrum.

DU-27 (Duiduan 兑端)

Indications

Lip stiffness, swelling and pain of the gum, mental disorders.

Location

At the junction of the lower end of the philtrum and the upper lip.

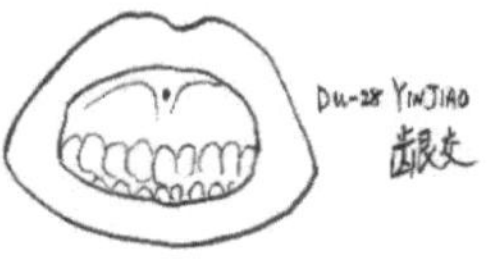

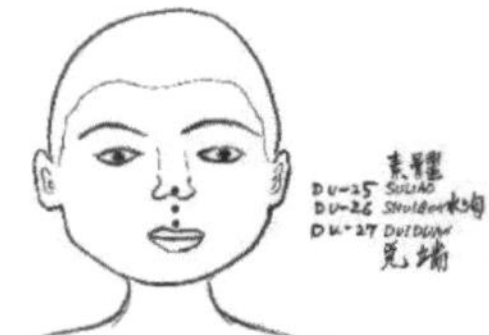

DU-28 (Yinjiao 龈交)

Indications

Swelling and pain of the gum, mental disorders, rhinorrhea.

Location

Inside the upper lip, at the junction of the labial frenum and the upper gum.

The Conception Vessel
XIV.Point of the Ren Channel　任脉经穴

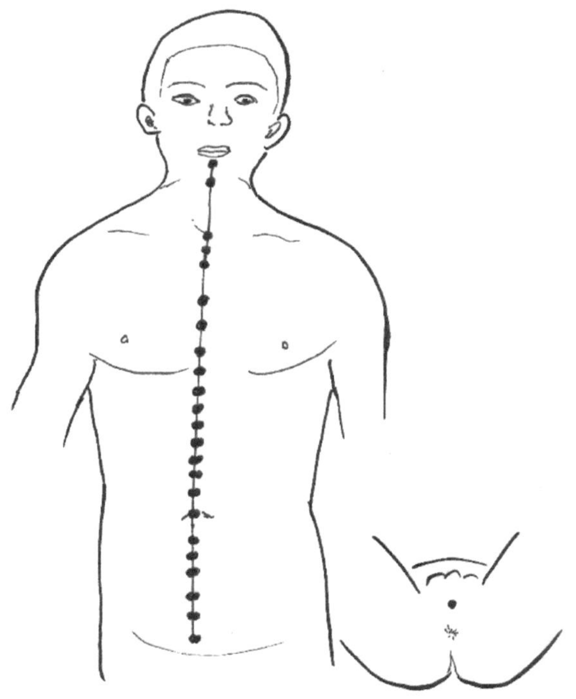

Starts above the middle of the pubic region and ascends straight up the middle of the body to below the lower lip. It contains 24 different acupoints.

REN-1 (Huiyin 会阴)
Indications

Hemorrhoids, nocturnal emission, enuresis, irregular menstruation, vaginitis, mental disorders.

Location

On the perineum, between the anus and the root of the serotum in males and between the anus and posterior labial commissure in females.

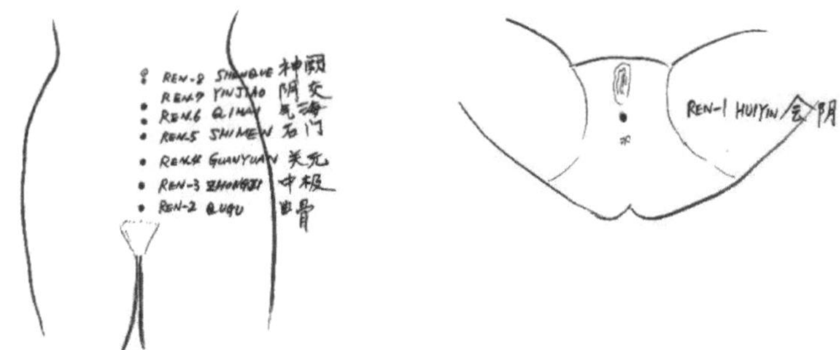

REN-2 (Qugu 曲骨)

Indications

Irregular menstruation, dysmenorrhea, leukorrhea, enuresis, unsmooth urination, impotence, seminal emission.

Location

On the lower abdomen, on the anterior midline, at the midpoint of the upper border of the pubic symphysis.

REN-3 (Zhongji 中极)

- **Front-Mu point of the Bladder.**

Indications

Irregular menstruation, metrorrhagia, dysmenorrhea, hernia, enuresis, prolapse of uterus, impotence, seminal emission, pain in the lower abdomen.

154

Location

On the lower abdomen, 4 cun below the umbilicus.

REN-4 (Guanyuan 关元)

- **Front-Mu point of the Small Intestine.**

Indications

Irregular menstruation, diarrhea, leukorrhea, frequent urination, seminal emission, hernia, impotence, hemorrhage, abdominal pain, emaciation.

Location

On the lower abdomen, 3 cun below the umbilicus.

REN-5 (Shimen 石门)

- **Front-Mu point of the Sanjiao.**

Indications

Abdominal pain, edema, diarrhea, edema, leukorrhea, amenorrhea, unsmooth urination, hernia, metrorrhagia.

Location

On the lower abdomen, 2 cun below the umbilicus.

REN-6 (Qihai 气海)

- **Sea of Qi.**

Indications

Abdominal pain, diarrhea, constipation, hernia, enuresis, irregular menstruation, amenorrhea, dysmenorrhea, apoplexy, asthma, nocturnal emission, impotence, edema.

Location

On the lower abdomen, 1.5 cun below the umbilicus.

REN-7 (Yinjiao 阴交)

Indications

Abdominal pain and distention, edema, hernia, irregular menstruation.

Location

On the lower abdomen, 1 cun below the umbilicus.

REN-8 (Shenque 神阙)

Indications

Abdominal pain, diarrhea, edema, prolapse of the rectum.

Location

In the centre of the umbilicus.

REN-9 (Shuifen 水分)

Indications

Abdominal pain, vomiting, regurgitation, edema, retention of urine, anuria.

Location

In the upper abdomen, 1 cun above the umbilicus.

REN-10 (Xiawan 下脘)

Indications

Abdominal pain and distension, vomiting, borborygmus, indigestion.

Location

On the upper abdomen, 2 cun above the umbilicus.

REN-11 (Jianli 建里)

Indications

Abdominal distention, borborygmus, edema, poor appetite.

Location

On the upper abdomen, 3 cun above the umbilicus.

REN-12 (Zhongwan 中脘)

- **Front-Mu point of the Stomach.**

Indications

Abdominal distention, stomachpain, borborygmus, hiccup, vomiting, acid regurgitation, edema, anorexia, diarrhea, insomnia, asthma.

Location

On the upper abdomen, 4 cun above the umbilicus.

REN-13 (Shangwan 上脘)

Indications

Stomachache, vomiting, abdominal distention, epilepsy.

Location

On the upper abdomen, 5 cun above the umbilicus.

REN-14 (Juqueju 巨阙)

- **Front-Mu point of the Heart.**

Indications

Pin in the chest and the cardiac region, vomiting, regurgitation, hiccup, epilepsy, palpitation, mental disorders.

Location

On the upper abdomen, 6 cun above the umbilicus.

REN-15 (Jiuwei 鸠尾)

- **Luo-Connecting point of the Conception vessel.**

Indications

Pain in the cardiac region, palpitation, dysphoria, depression, mania, jaundice, diarrhea, epilepsy.

Location

On the upper abdomen, 7 cun above the umbilicus, 1 cun below the sternocostal angle.

REN-16 (Zhongting 中庭)

Indications

Full and distention in the chest, hiccup, nausea, anorexia.

Location

On the chest, on the middle of the sternocostal angle.

REN-17(Shanzhong 膻中)

- **Front-Mu point of the Pericardium.**

Indications

Cough, asthma, chest pain, palpitation, angina pectoris, dysphoria, insomnia, breast abscess, insufficiency of lactation.

Location

At the level of the fourth intercostal space, the midpoint of the line connecting both nipples.

REN-18 (Yutang 玉堂)

Indications

Cough, asthma, chest pain, vomiting.

Location

On the midline of the chest, at the level of the third intercostal space.

REN-19 (Zigong 紫宫)

Indications

Pain in the chest, asthma, cough.

Location

On the midline of the chest, at the level of the second intercostal space.

REN-20 (Huagai 华盖)

Indications

Asthma, cough, pain in the chest and intercostal region.

Location

On the midline of the chest, at the level of the first intercostal space.

REN-21 (Xuanji 璇玑)

Indications

Cough asthma, chest pain, sore throat.

Location

On the chest, in the centre of the sternal manubrium, 1 cun posterior to REN-22 (Tiantu 天突).

REN-22 (Tiantu 天突)

Indications

Cough, asthma, chest pain, sore throat, dry throat, hiccup, loss of voice, goiter, dysphagia.

Location

On the neck, in the centre of the suprasternal fossa.

REN-23 (Lianquan 廉泉)

Indications

Aphasia due to stiff tongue, hoarseness of the voice, difficulty in swallowing, sublingual swelling and pain.

Location

On the neck, on the anterior midline, in the depression above the hyoid bone.

REN-24 (Chengjiang 承浆)

Indications

Swelling and pain of gum, deviation of the eyes and mouth, facial puffiness, epilepsy, mental disorders.

Location

On the face, in the depression at the midpoint of the mentolabial groove.

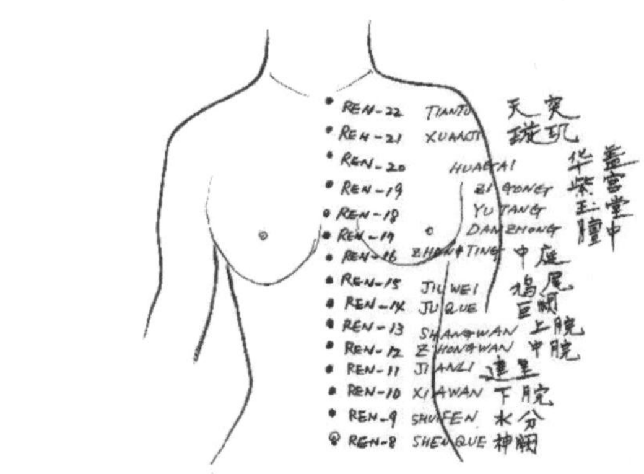

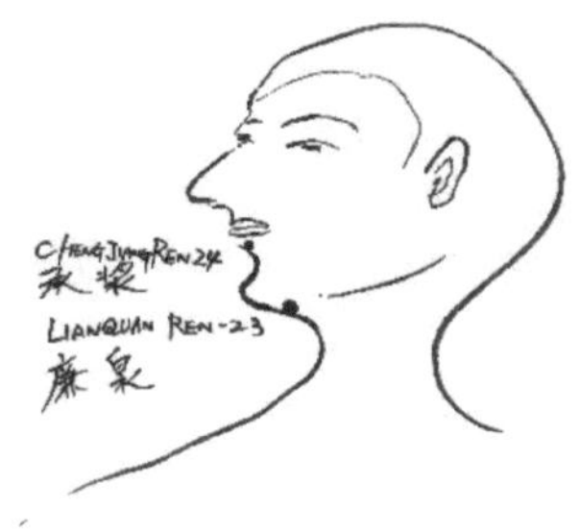

Section 4 Location of the Extra-ordinary Point 常用经外奇穴定位

(1). Points of the Head and Neck 头颈部穴

EX-HN1 Sishencong 四神聪

Indications

Headache, dizziness, insomnia, poor memory, epilepsy.

Location

Four points on the head 1 cun respectively, anterior and lateral to DU-20 (Baihui 白会).

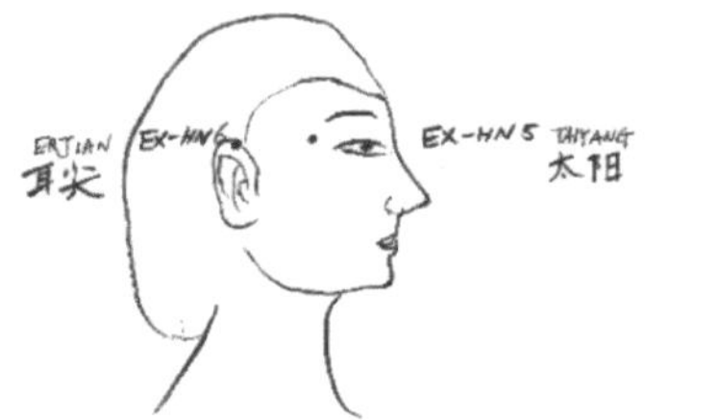

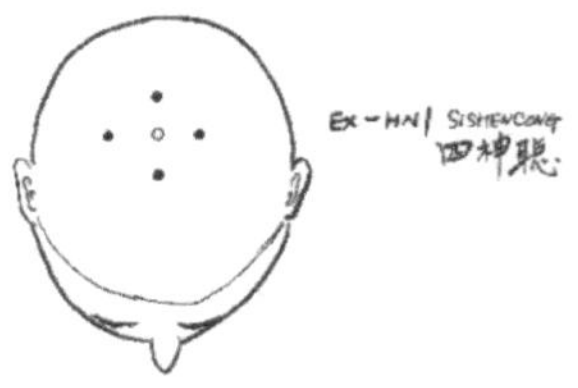

EX-HN2 Dangyang 当阳

Indications

Frontal headache, insomnia, poor memory.

Location

At the front part of the head, directly above the pupil, 0.5 cun above GB-15 (Toulinqi 头临泣).

EX-HN3 Yintang 印堂

Indications

Frontal headache, rhinorrhea, infantile convulsion.

Location

On the forehead, at the midpoint between the two eyebrows.

EX-HN4 Yuyao 鱼腰

Indications

Headache, rhinorrhea, frontal headache, insomnia, infantile convulsion.

Location

On the forehead, directly above the pupil, in the centre of the eyebrow.

EX-HN5 Taiyang 太阳

Indications

Headache, swelling and pain of the eye.

Location

At the temporal part of the head, in the depression 1 cun posterior to the midpoint between the lateral end of the eyebrow and the outer canthus of the eye.

EX-HN6 Erjian 耳尖

Indications

Swelling, redness and pain of the eyes, febrile disease.

Location

When the ear is folded forward, the point is located at the apex of the ear.

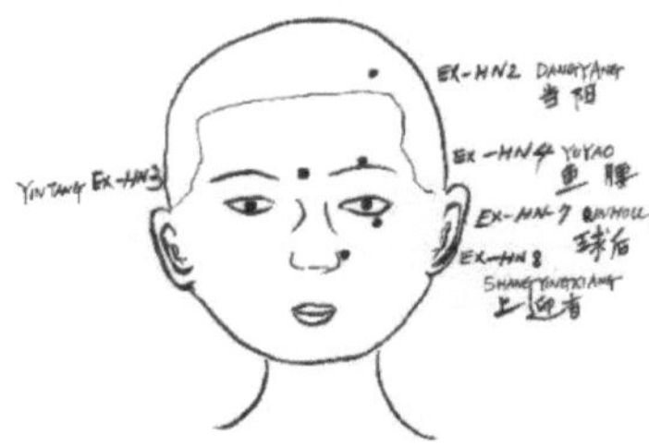

EX-HN7 Qiuhou 球后

Indications

Eye diseases.

Location

On the face, at the junction of the lateral fourth and medial three fourths of the infraorbital margin.

EX-HN8 Shangyingxiang 上迎香

Indications

Rhinorrhea, nasal obstruction.

Location

On the face, at the upper end of the nasolabial groove.

EX-HN9 Neiyingxiang 内迎香

Indications

Rhinorrhea, nasal obstruction.

Location

In the nostril, at the junction between the alar cartilage of the nose and the nose concha.

EX-HN10 Juquan 聚泉

Indications

Swelling and pain of the tongue, facial paralysis.

Location

In the mouth, at the midpoint of the midline on the tongue surface.

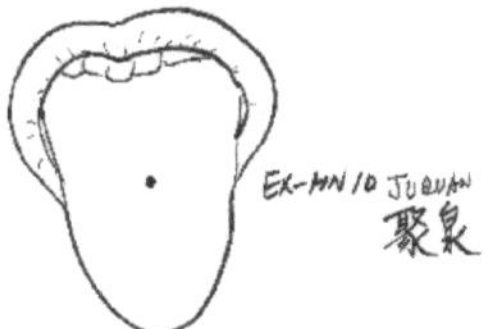

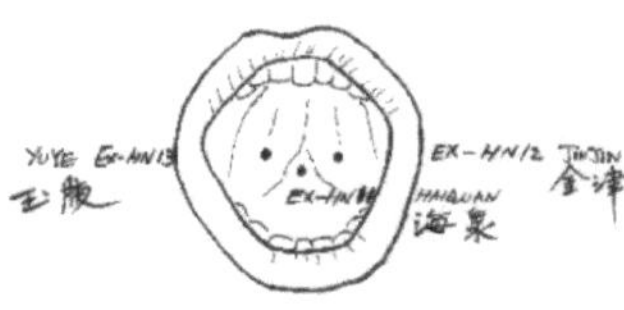

EX-HN11 Haiquan 海泉

Indications

Swelling and pain of the tongue, facial paralysis.

Location

At the midpoint of the frenulum of the tongue, between EX-HN12 Jinjin and EX-HN13 Yuye.

EX-HN12 Jinjin 金津

Indications

Swelling of the tongue, vomiting, stiffness of tongue due to aphasia.

Location

In the mouth, on the vein of the left side of the frenulum of the tongue.

EX-HN13 Yuye 玉腋

Indications

Swelling of the tongue, vomiting, stiffness of the tongue due to aphasia.

Location

In the mouth, on the vein of the right side of the frenulum of the tongue.

EX-HN14 Yiming 翳明

Indications

Eye diseases, tinnitus, insomnia.

Location

1 cun posterior to SJ-17 (Yifeng 翳风).

EX-HN15 Jingbailao 颈百劳

Indications

Cough, asthma, neck rigidity, scrofula.

Location

2 cun above DU-14 (Dazhui 大椎), 1 cun lateral to the midline.

EX-HN16 Anmian 安眠

Indications

Insomnia, headache, palpitation, vertigo, mental disorders.

Location

Behind the ear, between GB-20 (Fengchi 风池) and SJ-17 (Yifeng 翳风).

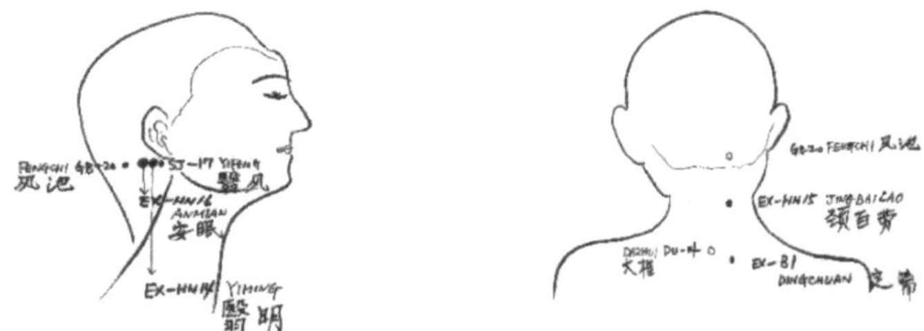

(2) Points of the Chest and Abdomen 胸腹部穴

EX-CA1 Zigong 子宫

Indications

Prolapse of the uterus, irregular menstruation.

Location

On the lower abdomen, 3 cun lateral to REN-3 (Zhongji 中极).

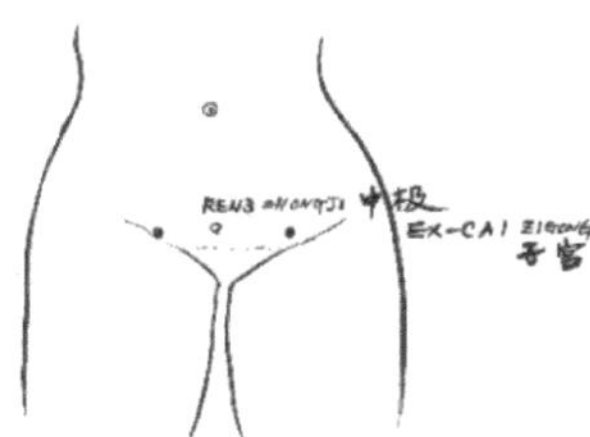

(3) Points of the Back 背部穴

EX-B1 Dingchuan 定喘

Indications

Asthma, cough, pain in the shoulder and neck.

Location

On the back, 0.5 cun lateral to DU-14 (Dazhui 大椎).

EX-B2 Jiaji 夹脊

Indications

Intercostal neuralgia, disease of spine.

Location

On each side of the back, 0.5 cun lateral to the lower border of each spinous process from the first thoracic vertebra to the fifth lumbar vertebra, totaling 17 points on each side.

EX-B3 Weiwanxiashu 胃脘下俞

Indications

Pain in the back, thirsting due to diabetes.

Location

On the back, below the spinous process of the eighth thoracic vertebra, 1.5 cun lateral to the posterior midline.

EX-B4 Pigen 痞根

Indications

Lumbar pain, hepatosplenomegaly.

Location

On the lower back, below the spinous process of the first lumbar vertebra, 3.5 cun lateral to the posterior midline.

EX-B5 Xiajishu 下极俞

Indications

Pain in the lower back.

Location

On the midline of the lower back, below the spinous process of the third lumber vertebra.

EX-B6 Yaoyi 腰宜

Indications

Epilepsy, headache, constipation, insomnia.

Location

On the lower back, below the spinous process of the fourth lumbar vertebra, 3 cun lateral to the posterior midline.

EX-B7 Yaoyan 腰眼

Indications

Pain in the lower back, pain of the lumbar.

Location

On the lower back, below the spinous process of the fourth lumbar vertebra, 3.5 cun lateral to the posterior midline.

EX-B8 Shiqizhui 十七椎

Indications

Lumbar and thigh pain, paralysis of the lower extremities, irregular menstruation, dysmenorrhea.

Location

On the lower back, the posterior midline below the spinous process of the fifth lumbar vertebra.

EX-B9 Yaoqi 腰奇

Indications

Headache, insomnia, epilepsy, constipation.

Location

On the lower back, 2 cun directly above the tip of the coccyx, in the depression between the sacral horns.

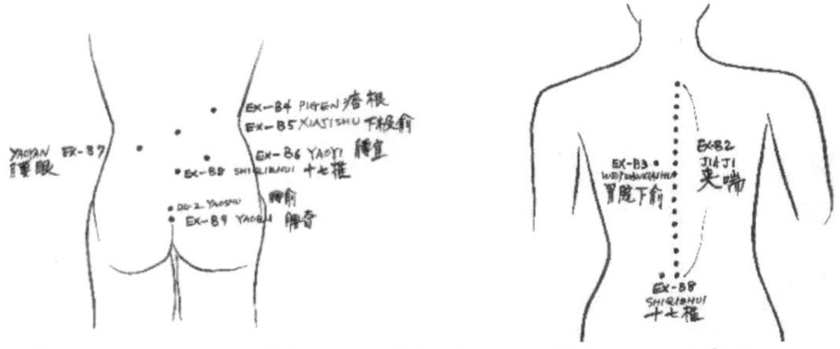

(4) Points on the Upper Extremities 上肢穴

EX-UE1 Zhoujian 肘尖

Indications

Scrofula

Location

On the posterior side of the elbow, at the tip of the ulnar olecranon when the elbow is flexed.

EX-UE2 Erbai 二白

Indications

Hemorrhoids, prolapse of the rectum.

Location

On the palmer side of forearm, a pair of points, 4 cun above the transverse crease of the wrist, on both sides of the tendon of m. flexor carpi radialis, two points on the hand.

EX-UE3 Zhongquan 中泉

Indications

Stuffy chest, gastric pain.

Location

On the dorsal crease of the wrist, in the depression on the radial side of the tendon of the m. extensor digitorum communis.

EX-UE4 Zhongkui 中魁

Indications

Nausea, hiccup, vomiting.

Location

On the dorsal side of the middle finger, at the center of the proximal interphalangeal joint.

EX-UE5 Dagukong 大骨空

Indications

Pain of the thumb, spasm, numbness of the little finger.

Location

On the dorsal side of the thumb, at the center of the interphalangeal joint.

EX-UE6 Xiaogukong 小骨空

Indications

Pain of the little finger, spasm, numbness of the little finger.

Location

On the dorsal side of the little finger, at the midpoint of the proximal interphalangeal joint.

EX-UE7 Yaotongdian 腰痛点

Indications

Lumbar sprain.

Location

On the dorsum of the hand, midway between the transverse crease of the wrist and the metacarpophalangeal joint, between the second and third metacarpal bones, between the fourth and fifth metacarpal bones, two points on each hand.

EX-UE8 Wailaogong 外劳宫

Indications

Cardiac pain, epilepsy, heart pain.

Location

On the dorsum of the hand, between second and third metacarpal bones.

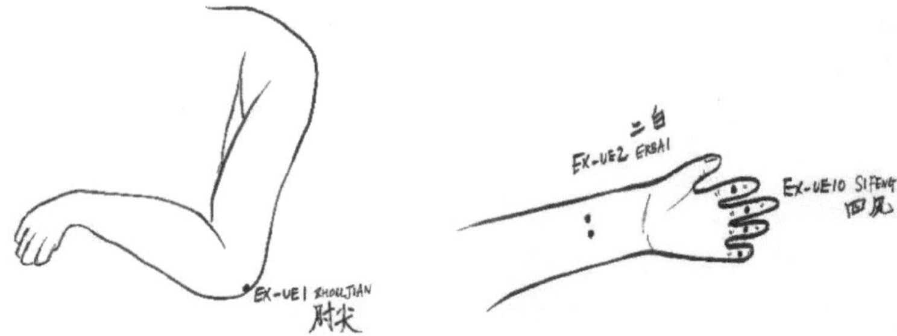

EX-UE9 Baxie 八邪

Indications

Spasm, numbness, of the fingers, swelling and pain of the dorsum of the hand.

Location

When the hand is made into a fist, the points are located at the ends of the vertical skin crease of the webs between every two fingers.

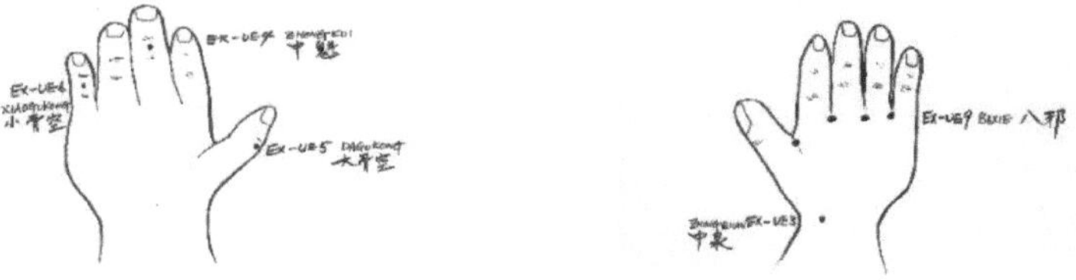

EX-UE10 Sifeng 四缝

Indications

Whooping cough, indigestion syndrome in children.

Location

On the palmar side of the hand, in the midpoint of the transverse crease of the proximal interphalangeal joint of the index, middle, ring and small fingers.

EX-UE11 Shixuan 十宣

Indications

Numbness of fingertips, apoplexy, high fever, coma, tonsilitis, epilepsy.

Location

On the tips of the ten fingers, 0.1cun distal to the nails.

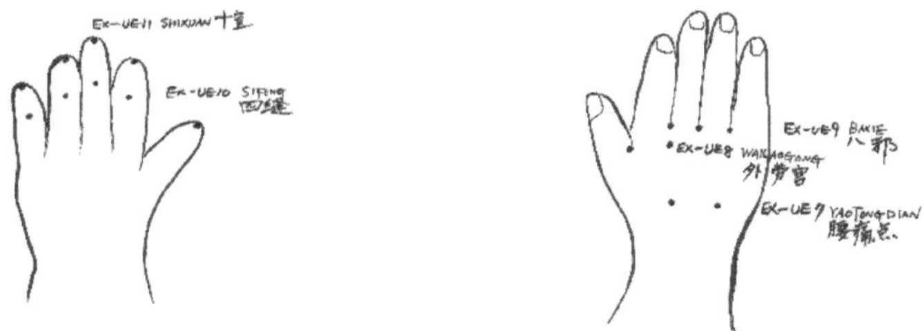

(5) Points on the Lower Extremities 下肢穴

EX-LE1 Kuangu 髋骨

Indications

Pain and numbness of the knee, paralysis.

Location

On the lower part of the anterior thigh, 1.5 cun lateral to ST-34 (Liang 梁丘), two points on each thigh.

EX-LE2 Heding 鹤顶

Indications

Knee pain, weakness of the foot and leg, paralysis.

Location

Above the knee, in the depression of the midpoint of the upper border of the patella.

EX-LE3 Baichongwo 百虫窝

Indications

Gastro-intestinal parasitic diseases, eczema.

Location

3 cun above the superior border of the patella, 1 cun above SP-10 (Xuehai 血海).

EX-LE4 Xiyan 膝眼

Indications

Knee pain, weakness of the lower extremities.

Location

When the knee is flexed, in the depression medial and lateral side of the patellar ligament, the medial side is called Neixiyan 内膝眼, on the lateral side is called Waixiyan 外膝眼.

EX-LE5 Dannang 胆囊

Indications

Muscular atrophy and numbness of the lower extremities, cholecystitis.

Location

At the upper part of the lateral of the leg, 2 cun below GB-34 (Yanglingquan 阳陵泉).

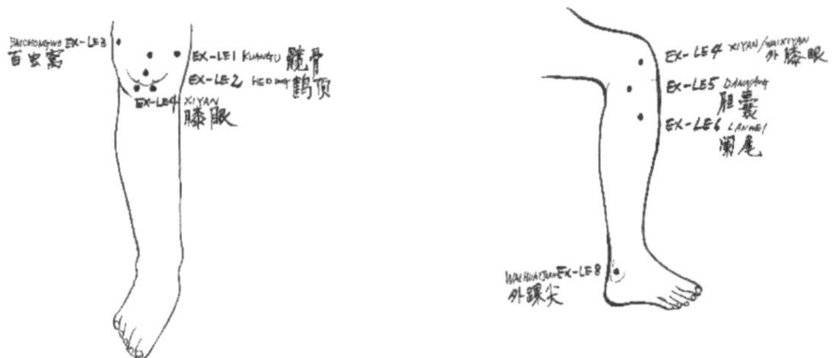

EX-LE6 Lanwei 阑尾

Indications

Apendicitis, paralysis of the lower extremities.

Location

At the upper part of the anterior of the leg, 2cun below ST-36 (Zusanli 足三里).

EX-LE7 Neihuaijian 内踝尖

Indications

Pain and paralysis of the lower extremities, muscular atrophy.

Location

On the medial side of the foot, at the prominence of the medial malleolus.

EX-LE8 Waihuaijian 外踝尖

Indications

Pain and paralysis of the lower extremities, muscular atrophy.

Location

On the lateral side of the foot, at the prominence of the lateral malleolus.

EX-LE9 Bafeng 八风

Indications

Toe pain, redness and swelling of the dorsum of the foot, numbness of the lower limb.

Location

On the dorsum of the foot, at the margin of the webs between each two toes, four points on each foot, eight points in all.

EX-LE10 Duyin 独阴

Indications

Pain, redness and swelling of the foot, muscular atrophy, pain, and numbness of the lower limb.

Location

On the plantar side of the second toe, at the midpoint of the transverse crease.

EX-LE11 Qiduan 气端

Indications

Pain, redness and swelling of the foot, muscular atrophy, numbness of the lower limb.

Location

On the tip of the ten toes, 0.1 cun distal to the nails, ten points in all.

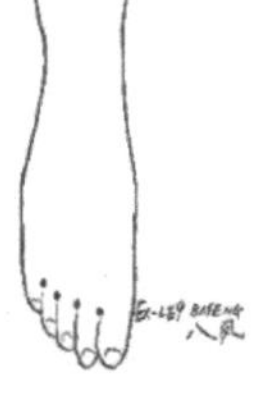

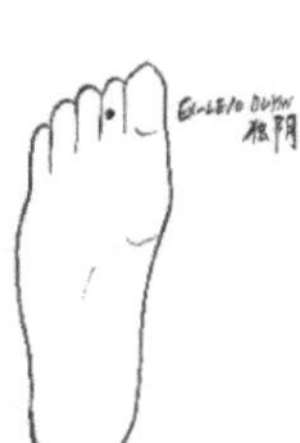

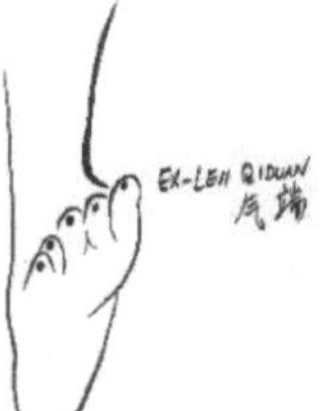

CHARPTER 3
Clinical Treatment of Common Diseases
A1. Internal Medicine

1-1 Abdominal Pain 腹痛 Futong

- **Differentiation**

1. Internal accumulation of cold:
   Sudden violent pain which responds to warmth and is aggravated by cold. Other manifestations include loose stools, profuse clear urine, white coated tongue, deep tense or deep slow pulse.

2. Retention of food:
   Epigastric and abdominal distension and pain which may be aggravated by pressure, foul belching and acidity. Abdominal pain may be accompanied by diarrhea and relieved after defecation. The tongue is sticky coated, the pulse is rolling.

- **Treatment**
  Prescription
  1.Accumulation of Cold in the interior
  REN-12 (Zhongwan 中脘), REN-8 (Shenque 神闕), ST-36 (Zusanli 足三里)

  2.Retention of food
  REN-10 (Xianwan 下脘), ST-21 (Liangmen 梁門), (Gongsun 公孫), ST-36 (Zusanli 足三里)

  3.Deficiency of Spleen Yang

BL-20 (Pishu 脾俞), BL-21 (Weishu 胃俞), REN-12 (Zhongwan 中脘), REN-4 （Guanyuan 关元）, REN-6 (Qihai 气海), LIV-13 (Zhangmen 章门)

- **Addition**
Pain above the umbilicus:
REN-10 (Xiawan 下脘), ST-36 (Zusanli 足三里)

Pain around the umbilicus:
ST-25 (Tianshu 天枢), REN-6 (Qihai 气海)

Pain in the lower abdomen:
REN-4 (Guanyuan 关元), SP-6(Sanyinjiao 三阴交)

- **Remarks**
By acute and severe abdominal pain, it is necessary to have the strict observation of the patient, and other therapeutic measures should be taken.

1-2 Asthma 哮喘 Xiaochuan

- **Differentiation**

1.Wind-Cold in the Lung:
The main manifestations include difficult respiration, cough with shortness of breath and wheezing sound in the throat, dilute sputum of white colour, cold limbs without sweating, greyish facial complexion, white or white greasy tongue coating, and superficial tense or superficial slippery pulse. It may be accompanied by chills, fever, headache.

2. Phlegm-Heat Retention in the Lung:

The main manifestations include shallow breathing, strong and coarse voice, cough with thick yellow sputum, stuffy sensation in the chest and epigastric region. It is accompanied by fever, dryness of the mouth, thirst with desire for cold drinking, yellow greasy or sticky coating tongue and rapid slippery pulse.

- **Treatment**

1. Wind-Cold in the lung:
   Prescription:
   LU-7 (Lieque 列缺), BL-13 (Feishu 肺俞), BL-12 (Fengmen 风门), ST-9 (Renying 人迎), EX-B1 (Dingchuan 定喘)

2. Phlegm-Heat Retention in the Lung:
   Prescription: LU-5 (Chize 尺泽), LU-6 (Kongzui 孔最), DU-14 (Dazhui 大椎), ST-40 (Fenglong 丰隆), LI-4 (Hegu 合谷), REN-17 (Danzhong 膻中)

1-3 BI Syndrome 痹症 Bizheng
- **Differentiation**

The main symptom is arthralgia, including soreness and numbness in the body limbs, joints and muscles, particularly in the wrist joints, elbow, knee and ankle areas. In prolonged cases, contracture of the extremities, or even swelling or deformity of joints may occur.

- **Treatment**

Prescriptin: Based on diseased/pain area.
Shoulder:
LI-15 (Jianyu 肩髃), SJ14 (Jianliao 肩髎), SI-10(Naoshu 臑俞), LI-4 (Hegu 合谷)

Elbow:
LI-11 (Quchi 曲池), SJ-10 (Tianjing 天井), LU-5(Chize 尺泽), SJ-5 (Waiguan 外关)

Wrist:
LI-5 (Yangxi 阳溪), SJ-4 (Yangchi 阳池), SJ-5 (Waiguan 外关), SI-4 (Wangu 腕骨)
Hip:
GB-30 (Huantiao 环跳), GB-29 (Juliao 居髎), GB-39 (Xuanzhong 悬钟)

Knee:
ST-34 (Liangqiu 梁丘), SP-10 (Xuehai 血海), SP-9 (Yinlingquan 阴陵泉), GB-34 (Yanglingquan 阳陵泉), EX-LE4 (Xiyan 膝眼)

Ankle:
ST-41 (Jiexi 解溪), SP-5 (Shangqiu 商丘), BL-60(Kunlun 昆仑), KI-3 (Taixi 太溪), GB-40 (Qiuxu 丘墟)

Lumbar region:
DU-3 (Yaoyangguan 腰阳关), DU-12 (Shenzhu 身柱), DU-14 (Dazhui 大椎), EX-B1 (jiaji 夹脊)

- **Remarks**

BI syndrome may be seen in rheumatic fever, rheumatic arthritis, and rheumatoid arthritis.

- **Moxibution**
  REN-8 (Shenque 神阙) with ginger slice with small holes may apply.

1-4 Back Pain 背痛 Beitong

- **Differentiation**

  The exogenous factor mainly refers to the pathogenic wind-cold invading, causing blockage in the meridians, Qi and Blood circulation, and becomes back pain.

- **Treatment**
  Prescription:
  DU-14 (Dazhui 大椎), DU-12 (Shenzhu 身柱), Du-9 (Zhiyang 至阳), Extra (Jiaji 夹脊), Ashi point, BL-40 (Weizhong 委中), BL-60 (Kunlun 昆仑)

1-5 Common Cold 普通感 Putongganmao

- **Differentiation**
1. Wind-Cold Type
   Mild fever without sweating, aversion to cold, headache, running nose, cough, thin whitish Sputum, thin white tongue coating, rapid superficial pulse.

2. Wind-Heat Type
High fever, spontaneous sweating, headache, stuffy nose, sore throat, dry mouth with desire for drinking, cough with yellowish thick sputum, thin yellow tongue coating, rapid superficial pulse.

3. Damp-Heat Type
The Main manifestations are high fever without sweating, headache, fullness sensation in the chest, lassitude, nausea, anorexia, abdominal distention, loose stool, sticky whitish sputum, thick yellow tongue coating, soft rapid pulse.

- **Treatment**
  Prescription
1. Wind-Cold Type
   LU-7 (Lieque 列缺), BL-12 (fengmen 风门), GB-20 (Fengchi 凤池), LI-4 (Hegu 合谷)
2. Wind-Heat Type
   LU-5 (Chize 尺泽), LU-10 (Yuji 鱼际), LI-4 (Hegu 合谷), LI-11 (Quchi 曲池), DU-14 Dazhui 大椎)
3. Damp-Heat type
   LU-6 (Kongzui 孔最), LI-4 (Hegu 合谷), REN-12 (Zhongwan 中脘), ST-36 (Zusanli 足三里), SJ-5 (Waiguan 外关)

1-6 Cough 咳嗽 Kesou

- **Differentiation**

1. Exopathogenic Factors
(1) Wind-Cold Type

It is characterized by itching sensation in the throat. It is accompanied by fever, chills, headache, nasal obstruction, soreness of joints. The tongue has thin white coating, and superficial pulse.

(2) Wind-Heat Type
Fever without chills, thirst, cough with thick sputum, dry mouth and sticky yellowish sputum, tongue with yellowish coating, rapid superficial pulse.

2. Endopathogenic Factors
(1) Yang Deficiency with Spleen
Cough with excessive sputum, fullness sensation in the chest and epigastric region, listlessness, white greasy tongue coating, deep and slow pulse.

(2) Yin Deficiency with Dryness of the Lung
Dry cough without sputum, dry throat, feverish palms and soles, fever, red tongue with thin coating, feeble rapid pulse.

- **Treatment**
  Prescription:
1. Exopathogenic Factors
(1) Wind-Cold Type
LU-7 (Lieque 列缺), LI-4 (Hegu 合谷), BL-13 (Feishu 肺俞), SJ-5 (Waiguan 外关)
(2) Wind-Heat Type
LU-5 (Chize 尺泽), LI-11 (Quchi 曲池), DU-14 (Dazhui 大椎), BL-13 (Feishu 肺俞)

2. Endopathogenic Factors

(1) Yang Deficiency with Spleen
   LU-9 (Taiyuan 太渊), SP-3 (Taibai 太白), ST-40 (Fenglong 丰隆), BL-13 (Feishu 肺俞), BL-20 (Pishu 脾俞)

(2) Yin Deficiency with Dryness of the Lung
   LU-1 (Zhongfu 中府), LU-7 (Lieque 列缺), BL-13 (Feishu 肺俞), KI-6 (Zhaohai 照海), LIV-3 (Taichong 太冲)

1-7 Constipation 便秘 Bianmi

- **Differentiation**

1. Heat Type
   Absence of bowel motions for several days, abdominal pain, fullness and distention, restlessness, dry mouth with foul breath, yellow tong coating, rapid slippery pulse.

2. Qi Stagnation Type
   Frequent bowel movements, distending pain in the abdomen, bitter taste, dizziness, poor appetite, thin greasy tongue coating, thready pulse.

3. Deficient Type
   Dry stool difficult to discharge, shortness of breath and lassitude, no distention and pain of abdomen, palpitation, dizziness, blurred vision, pale tongue, thin coating, thin feeble pulse.

4. Cold Type

Dry stool difficult to discharge, occasional pain of abdomen, cold limbs, clear urine, pale tongue with white coating, deep slow pulse.

- **Treatment**

Prescription

1. Heat Type
   LI-4 (Hegu 合谷), LI-11 (Quchi 曲池), ST-25 tianshu 天枢), ST-44 (Neiting 内庭), SP-14 (Fujie 腹结), ST-37 (Shangjuxu)

2. Qi Stagnation Type
   REN-12 (Zhongwan 中脘), ST-25 (Tianshu 天枢), GB-34 (Yanglingquan 阳陵泉), SJ-6 (Zhigou 支沟), LIV-2 (Xingjian 行间)

3. Deficient Type
   REN-4 (Guanyuan 关元), REN-6 (Qihai 气海), BL-20 (Pishu 脾俞), BL-21 (Weishu 胃俞), ST-36 (Zusanli 足三里)

4. Cold Type
   REN-6 (Qihai 气海), REN-8 (Shenque 神阙), ST-25 (Tianshu 天枢), KI-6 (Zhaohai 照海), BL-23 (Shenshu 肾俞)

1-8 Diarrhea 泄泻 Xiexie

- **Differenciation**

1. Acute Diarrhea
(1) Cold-Damp Type

Loose stools with abdominal pain, borborygmus, cold with desire for warmth, absence of thirst, pale tongue with white coating, deep and slow pulse.

(2) Damp-Heat Type

Loose stools with abdominal pain, urgent bowel motion, feverish sensation in the anus, scanty urine, yellow greasy tongue coating, rapid slippery soft pulse.

2. Chronic Diarrhea

(1) Spleen Yang Deficiency

Loose stools with undigested food, abdominal and epigastric distension, anorexia, lassitude, white sticky tongue coating, soft slow pulse.

(2) Kidney Yang Deficiency

Abdominal pain, borborygmus and diarrhea before dawn, cold extremities, white tongue coating, deep forceless pulse.

- **Treatment**

Prescription

1. Acute Diarrhea

(1) Cold-Damp type

ST-25 (Tianshu 天枢), ST-37 (Shangjuxu 上巨虚), REN-6 (Qihai 气海), REN-11 (Jianli 建里), SP-9 (Yinlingquan 阴陵泉)

(2)   Damp-Heat Type

ST-44 (Neiting 内庭), ST-25 (Tianshu 天枢), REN-12 (Zhongwan 中脘), SP-9 (Yinlingquan 阴陵泉), LI-11 (Quchi 曲池)

2. Chronic Diarrhea
(1) Spleen Yang Deficiency
SP-3 (Taibai 太白), ST-25 (Tianshu 天枢), ST-36 (Zusanli 足三里), BL-20 (Pishu 脾俞), REN-12 (Zhongwan 中脘), LIV-13 (Zhangmen 章门)
(2) Kidney Yang Deficiency
BL-20 (Pishu 脾俞), BL-23 (Shenshu 肾俞), DU-4 (Mingmen 命门), REN-4 (Guanyuan 关元), ST-25 (Tianshu 天枢), ST-37 (Shangjuxu 上巨虚)

1-9 Dizziness 眩晕 Xuanyun

- **Differentiation**

1. Hyperactivity of Liver Yang
The manifestations are tinnitus, nausea, backache disturbed sleep, flushed face, congested eyes, red tongue proper with thin yellow coating, wiry rapid pulse.
2. Qi and Blood Deficiency
The manifestations are palpitation, insomnia, pale complexion, poor appetite, pale tongue proper, weak pulse.
3. Phlegm-Damp obstruction in the interior
The manifestations are lassitude, fullness in the chest and epigastrium, heaviness of head, vomiting, white and sticky tongue, rolling pulse.

- **Treatment**

Prescription
1. Hyperactivity of Liver Yang
GB-20 (Fengchi 凤池), GB-43 (Xiaxi 侠溪), LIV-3 (Taichong 太冲), BL-18 (Ganshu 肝俞)

2. Qi and Blood Deficiency
   BL-20 (Pishu 脾俞), BL-23 (Shenshu 肾俞), ST-36 (Zusanli 足三里), SP-6 (Sanyinjiao 三阴交), REN-4 (Guanyuan 关元), DU-20 (Baihui 百会)

3. Phlegm-Damp obstruction in the interior
   REN-12 (Zhongwan 中脘), DU-20 (Baihui 百会), BL-20 (Pishu 脾俞), P-6 (Neiguan 内关), ST-36 (Zusanli 足三里), ST-40 (Fenglong 丰隆)

1-10 Depressive Manic Mental Disorders 抑郁性燥狂症 Yiyuxingzaokuangzheng

- **Differentiation**
1. Depressive mental disorders
   Gradual onset, mental depression and dullness at the initial stage. It is followed by paraphasia, muteness, hypersomnia and anorexia, illusions. Tongue is thin greasy coating, and thready and wiry pulse.

2. Manic mental disorders
   Sudden onset proceeds by irritability, less sleep and no desire for eating. The manifestation followed by shouting, violent behavior, destroying the objects and harming people. Yellow greasy tongue coating, and rapid slippery pulse.

- **Treatment**
   Prescription
(1) Depressive mental disorders

BL-15 (Xinshu 心俞), BL-18 (Ganshu 肝俞), BL-20 (Pishu 脾俞), ST-40 (Fenglong 丰隆), HT-7 (Shenmen 神门), P-7 (Daling 大陵), REN-17 (Danzhong 膻中), LIV-3 (Taichong 太冲)

(2) Manic mental disorders
DU-14 (Dazhui 大椎), DU-16 (Fengfu 风府), DU-26 (Shuigou 水沟), P-5 (Jianshi 间使), P-8 (Laogong 劳宫), ST-40 (Fenglong 丰隆)

- **Remarks**
Depressive and Manic Mental Disorders corresponds to Bipolar in modern medicine.

1-11 Diabetes 糖尿病 Tangniaobing

- **Differentiation**
(1) Upper Diabetes
Thirst, dry mouth, profuse urination, polydipsia, red tip of the tongue, thin yellow tongue coating, full rapid pulse.

(2) Middle Diabetes
Polyphagia, easy hunger, restlessness, profuse sweating, emaciation, profuse drinking of water, polyuria, dry yellow tongue coating, slippery rapid pulse.

(3) Lower Diabetes
Profuse and frequent urination, turbid urine with sweet taste, thirst and polydipsia, dizziness, blurred vision, red cheeks, soreness and weakness of the knee, red tongue, thin and rapid pulse.

- **Treatment**
  Prescription
(1) Upper Diabetes
  HT-8 (Shaofu 少府), LU-9 (Taiyuan 太渊), BL-13 (Feishu 肺俞), BL-15 (Xinshu 心俞)

(2) Middle Diabetes
  BL-20 (Pishu 脾俞), BL-21 (Weishu 胃俞), ST-44 (Neiting 内庭), SP-6 (Sanyinjiao 三阴交)

(3) Lower Diabetes
  BL-18 (Ganshu 肝俞), KI-3 (Taixi 太溪), LIV-3 (Taichong 太冲), BL-23 (Shenshu 肾俞)

- **Remarks**
  Diabetes is characterized by polydipsia, polyphagia, polyuria, emaciation and sweet urine.

1-12 Edema 水肿 Shuizhong

- **Differentiation**
(1) Yang Edema
  It characterized by acute in nature, and firstly show puffiness of the face, eyelids, limbs. The skin is lustrous. It accompanies cough, asthma, fever, thirst, scanty urine, and lower back pain, superficial rapid pulse.
(2) Yin Edema
  It characterized by a slow onset, swelling face is the first stage, and then spreads to the abdomen and whole body.

When pressing on hand, appear rebound slowly. Symptoms are short urine, loose stools, lassitude, weak limbs, pale tongue with white coating, deep thready slow pulse.

- **Treatment**

Prescription
(1) Yang Edema
BL-13 (Feishu 肺俞), BL-22 (Sanjiaoshu 三焦俞), LI-6 (Pianli 偏历), LI-4 (Hegu 合谷), SJ-5 (Waiguan 外关), SP-9 (Yinlingquan 阴陵泉)

(2) Yin Edema
BL-20 (Pishu 脾俞), BL-23 (Shenshu 肾俞), ST-36 (Zusanli 足三里), REN-9 (Shuifen 水分), REN-6 (Qihai 气海), KI-3 (Taixi 太溪)

- **Remarks**
Edema refers to retention of fluid in the body and shows puffiness of the head, face, eyelids, limbs, whole body.

1-13 Epigastric Pain 上腹痛 Shangfutong

- **Differentiation**
1. Attack on stomach by Liver Qi
(1) Qi Stagnation
Epigastric pain, distending pain in the hypochondriac region, nausea, deep and wiry pulse, thin white tongue coating.

(2) Stagnant Heat

Sudden onset of epigastric pain, restlessness, irritability, dry mouth, discomfort sensation of stomach, red and yellow coating tongue, rapid thready pulse.

(3) Blood Stasis

Pain, aggravated by food and pressing, vomiting, dark purplish tongue, uneven pulse.

2. Retention of Food

Distention and pain in the epigastric region, belching, acid regurgitation, pain aggravated after food intake, thick greasy tongue coating, deep slippery pulse.

3. Deficient Cold in the Spleen and Stomach

The manifestations are dull pain in the epigastric area, and relieved by warmth and pressing, listlessness, cold limbs, loose stools, pale tongue, weak pulse.

- **Treatment**

Prescription

1. Attack on stomach by Liver Qi

(1) Qi Stagnation

LIV-14 (Qimen 期门), ST-36 (Zusanli 足三里), REN-12 (Zhongwan 中脘), P-6 (Neiguan 内关), LIV-3 (Taichong 太冲)

(2) Stagnant Heat

REN-12 (Zhongwan 中脘), ST-36 (Zusanli 足三里), P-6 (Neiguan 内关), LIV-2 (Xingjian 行间), KI-3 (Taixi 太溪)

(3) Blood Stasis

REN-12 (Zhongwan 中脘), P-6 (Neiguan 内关), BL-17 (Geshu 膈俞), SP-4 (Gongsun 公孙), SP-10 (Xuehai 血海)

2. Retention of Food
ST-25 (Tianshu 天枢), ST-21 (Liangmen 梁门), ST-36 (Zusanli 足三里), REN-12 (Zhongwan 中脘)

3. Deficient Cold in the Spleen and Stomach
BL-20 (Pishu 脾俞), BL-21 (Weishu 胃俞), ST-36 (Zusanli 足三里), REN-12 (Zhongwan 中脘), LIV-13 (Zhangmen 章门)

1-14 Frozen Shoulder 肩周炎 Jianzhouyan
Shoulder Pain 肩痛 Jiantong

- **Differentiation**

Shoulder pain is named in TCM as frozen shoulder or fifty years old shoulder. The exogenous pathogenic wind, cold and damp overcome patients who are exhausted, overstrained, injured, and while sleeping in the shoulder.

Pain on shoulders alleviates in the daytime and worsens at night. It may involve back. It may aggravate with cold and alleviate with warmth.

- **Treatment**

LI-15 (Jianyu 肩髃), LI-11 (Quchi 曲池), LI-14 (Binao 臂臑), LI-4 (Hegu 合谷), SI-9 (Jianzhen 肩贞), SI-3 (Houxi 后溪), SJ-5 (Waiguan 外关)

- **Remarks**
  It is characterized by a heavy aching on shoulders, and it mostly appears to the person after fifty years old.

1-15 Hiccup 呃逆 Eni

- **Differentiation**

1. Retention of food and stagnation of Qi
   Epigastric and abdominal distension, sticky, yellow tongue coating, rolling forceful pulse.

2. Attack by pathogenic Cold
   Alleviated by hot drinks, white moist tongue coating, slow pulse.

- **Treatment**
  Prescription
  BL-17 (Geshu 膈俞), REN-12 (Zhongwan 中脘), REN-17 (Danzhong 膻中), P-6 (Neiguan 内关), ST-36 (Zusanli 足三里)

- **Remarks**

  It is mostly the result of adverse rise of Stomach Qi which is caused by the injury or blockage of overeating of raw and cold food.

1-16 Hypochondriac Pain 下软骨痛 Xiaruangutong

- **Differentiation**

(1) Stagnation of QI
Distending pain in hypochondrium, fullness sensation in the chest, irritability, thin white coating, wiry pulse.

(2) Stagnation of Blood
Fixed stabbing pain in the hypochondrium, pain worse by pressing, dark purplish tongue, wiry pulse.

- **Treatment**

Prescription
(1) Stagnation of QI
BL-18 (Ganshu 肝俞), Liv-3 (Taichong 太冲), Liv-14 (Qimen 期门), GB-34 (Yanglingquan 阳陵泉), SJ-6 (Zhigou 支沟)

(2)　Stagnation of Blood
BL-17 (Geshu 膈俞), BL-18 (Ganshu 肝俞), SP-6 (Sanyinjiao 三阴交), LIV-3 (Taichong 太冲), SJ-6 (Zhigou 支沟), LIV-14 (Qimen 期门)

- **Remarks**

Hypochondriac pain is caused from melancholy and anger which leads to the failure of Liver and QI.

1-17 Headache 头痛 Toutong

- **Differentiation**

Headache differentiation is according to its locality and channels. Pain at the occipital area and neck relate to Bladder channel. Pain at the forehead and supraorbital region relates to the Stomach channel, Pain at the temporal region of both sides and one side relates to the Gall Bladder channel. Pain at the parietal region relates to the Liver channel.

- **Treatment**
Prescription
1. Points according to the Headache region

(1) Occipital Headache
GB-20 (Fengchi 凤池), BL-60 (Kunlun 昆仑), SI-3 (Houxi 后溪)

(2) Frontside Headache
ST-8 (Touwei 头维), EX-HN5 (Yintang 印堂), LI-4 (Hegu 合谷)

(3) One-side Headache
GB-8 (Shuaigu 率谷), SJ-5 (Waiguan 外关), EX-HN5 (Taiyang 太阳)

(4) Parietal Headache
DU-20 (Baihui 百会), LIV-3 (Taichong 太冲), SI-3 (Houxi 后溪)

194

2. Points according to the symptoms and signs

(1) Hyperactivity of Yang of Liver
LIV-2 (Xingjian 行间), GB-34 (Yanglingquan 阳陵泉)

(2) Qi and Blood Deficiency
ST-36 (Zusanli 足三里), REN-6 (Qihai 气海)

1-18 Impotence 阳痿 **Yangwei**

- **Differentiation**
It is characterized by the penis inability and erection. The manifestation shows, dizziness, blurring vision, listlessness, poor sprit, frequent urination, weakness knee and lumbar region, insomnia, palpitation, Heart and Spleen may be involved.

- **Treatment**
Prescription
1. Declining QI
REN-4 (Guanyuan 关元), REN-3 (Zhongji 中极), KI-3 (Taixi 太溪), DU-20 (Baihui 百会), BL-23 (Shenshu 肾俞)

2. Declining Heat and Spleen QI
BL-15 (Xinshu 心俞), HT-7 (Shenmen 神门), SP-6 (Sanyinjiao 三阴交)

1-19 Insomnia 不寐 **Bumei**

- **Differentiation**

1. Heart and Spleen Deficiency
   Difficulty in falling asleep and disturbed sleep, palpitation, poor memory, poor appetite, loose stool, sallow complexion, thin white tongue coating, thready weak pulse.

2. Heart and Kidney Disharmony
   Insomnia accompanied by dizziness, tinnitus, leukorrhagia, feverish sensation in the palms and soles, red tongue with less coating, rapid weak pulse.

3. Liver Fire Disturbance
   Manifestations are dizziness, short temper, restlessness, hypochondriac pain, thin yellow tongue, wiry rapid pulse.

4. Stomach Dysfunction
   Insomnia accompanied by fullness in the epigastric region, abdominal distension, belching, acid regurgitation, yellow greasy tongue coating, wiry pulse.

- **Treatment**
  Prescription

1. Heart and Spleen Deficiency
   BL-20 (Pishu 脾俞), BL-15 (Xinshu 心俞), SP-1 (Yinbai 隐白), HT-7 (Shenmen 神门), SP-6 (Sanyinjiao 三阴交)

2. Heart and Kidney Disharmony
   BL-15 (Xinshu 心俞), BL-23 (Shenshu 肾俞), KI-3 (Taixi 太溪), HT-7 (Shenmen 神门), KI-6 (Zhaohai 照海)

196

3. Liver Fire Disturbance
   BL-18 (Ganshu 肝俞), LIV-3 (Taichong 太冲), LIV-2 (Xingjian 行间), HT-7 (Shenmen 神门)

4. Stomach Dysfunction
   BL-21 (Weishu 胃俞), ST-36 (Zusanli 足三里), REN-12 (Zhongwan 中脘), HT-7 (Senmen 神门)

1-20 Jaundice 黄疸 Huandan

- **Differentiation**

(1) Yang Type
   The Jaundice of Yang type is accompanied with fever, thirst, heavy sensation of the body, abdominal distention, fullness in the chest, nausea, yellow greasy tongue coating, wiry rapid pulse.
(2) Yin Type
   The Jaundice of Yin type is accompanied with heavy sensation of the body, and with slow over a long duration, nausea, vomiting, no thirst, tasteless, white greasy tongue coating, deep slow pulse.

- **Treatment**

   Prescription
(1) Yang Type
   LIV-3 (Taichong 太冲), GB-34 (Yanglingquan 阳陵泉), BL-18 (Ganshu 肝俞), DU-9 (Zhiyang 至阳), BL-19 (Danshu 胆俞), SI-4 (Wangu 腕骨)
(2) Yin Type

BL-20 (Pishu), SP-6 (Sanyinjiao 三阴交), ST-36 (Zusanli 足三里), REN-12 (Zhongwan 中脘), BL-19 (Danshu 胆俞), DU-9 (Zhiyang 至阳)

- **Remarks**
  Jaundice is characterized by yellow colour of sclera, and skin and urine. The bright yellow indicates Yang type and dark yellow indicates Yin type.

1-21 Lower Back Pain 下腰痛 **Xiayaotong**

- **Differentiation**

1. Cold-Damp
   Low back pain occurs often after invasion in pathogenic wind, cold and damp. The pain is characterized by a rapid onset of aching and soreness, stiffness of muscles, limiting extension and flexion of the back. The pain may lead downward to the buttocks and lower extremities that makes the patient feel difficult to bend forward and backward. Pain becomes worse in cloudy and rainy days. The tongue is white greasy, and the pulse is weak, deep and slow.

2. Kidney Deficiency
   Slow onset of hidden pain, in the lumber region in mild pain but protracted, weakness of the lumbar region and knee. Symptoms are intensified after strain and stress, white coating tongue, deep thready pulse.

3. Trauma

There is a traumatic history by patient. The manifestations are fixed local pain and rigidity, worsens by pressing and turning of the body, dark purplish tongue, wiry choppy pulse.

- **Treatment**
  Prescription
1. Cold-Damp
   BL-23 (Shenshu 肾俞), DU-3 (Yaoyanguan 腰阳关), BL-40 (Weizhong 委中)

2. Kidney Deficiency
   DU-4 (Mingmen 命门), KI-3 (Taixi 太溪), BL-23 (Shenshu 肾俞)
3. Trauma
   BL-17 (Geshu 膈俞), BL-40 (Weizhong 委中), BL-32 (Ciliao 次髎), Ashi points

- **Remarks**
  It involves the spine which one side or both sides of the lumbar. It refers to soft tissue injury, muscular rheumatism and lumbar disc degeneration.

1-22 Migrane 偏头痛 Piantoutong

- **Manifestation**
  Blurred vision, irritability, hot temper, red tongue with yellow coating, and string rapid pulse.
- **Differentiation**

(1) Pathogenic Wind Invasion

(2) Qi Stagnation due to Liver Yang upsurge
(3) Qi and Blood Deficiency

- **Treatment**

(1) One-side of the face
GB-8 (Shuaigu 率谷), SJ-5 (Waiguan 外关), EX-HN5 (Taiyang 太阳), ST-8 (Touwei 头维), EX-HN5 (Yintang 印堂), LI-4 (Hegu 合谷), ST-4 (Dicang 地仓)

(2) On Head
DU-20 (Baihui 百会), LIV-3 (Taichong 太冲), SI-3 (Houxi 后溪), EX-HN1 (Sishencong 四神聪), GB-20 (Fengchi 凤池), ST-8 (Touwei 头维), BL-7 (Tongtian 通天)

1-23 Nocturnal enuresis 遗尿 Yiniao

- **Differentiation**

It refers involuntary urination during sleep with dreams at night. It refers involuntary urinary discharge, and it is often seen in children, and it is also mostly seen in the aged patients.

1. Kidney Yang Deficiency
It happens during sleep, and the patient is not aware of it until waking up. The symptoms accompany with emaciation, lassitude, cold limbs, weak knee and lumber, pale tongue, deep slow pulse.

2. Lung and Spleen Qi Deficiency

There is frequent and hasty urine, and it accompanies with shortness of breath, lassitude, poor appetite, weakness of the limbs, loose stools, pale tongue slow, deep thready pulse.

3. Damp-Heat
Frequent urination, occasional enuresis, incontinence of urine, short scanty urine, dripping urine, lower fever, thin greasy tongue.

- **Treatment**
Prescription
1. Kidney Yang Deficiency
BL-28 (Pangguangshu 膀胱), REN-3 (Zhongji 中极), SP-6 (Sanyinjiao 三阴交), KI-3 (Taixi 太溪), BL-23 (Shenshu 肾俞), REN-4 (Guanyuan 关元)

2 Lung and Spleen Deficiency
LU-9 (Taiyuan 太渊), BL-13 (Feishu 肺俞), BL-20 (Pishu 脾俞), SP-6 (Sanyinjiao 三阴交), REN-6 (Qihai 气海), ST-36 (Zusanli 足三里)

3. Damp-Heat
SP-6 (Sanyinjiao 三阴交), SP-9 (Yinlingquan 阴陵泉), REN-3 (Zhongji 中极), BL-28 (Pangguangshu 膀胱俞), BL-39 (Weiyang 委阳)

4. Blood Stasis
SP-6 (Sanyinjiao 三阴交), BL-32 (Ciliao 次髎), REN-3 (Zhongji 中极), BL-17 (Geshu 膈俞), REN-6 (Qihai 气海)

- **Remarks**
Enuresis and incontinence are related to the function of Lower region, dysfunction of urinary bladder, which the urinary Bladder does not control urination.

1-24 Palpitation 心悸 Xinji

- **Differentiation**

1. Qi and Blood Insufficiency
The manifestations are lassitude, palpitation, pallor, disturbed sleep, pale tongue, weak thready pulse.

2. Plegm-Fire Disturbance
The manifestations are restlessness, dream-disturbed sleep, irritability, yellow urine, sticky sputum, yellow greasy tongue coating, rapid slippery pulse.

3. Blood Status
The manifestations are sallow emaciated complexion, palpitation, asthmatic breathing, cold limbs, thready, choppy pulse.

- **Treatment**
Prescription
1. Qi and Blood Insufficiency
BL-15 (Xinshu 心俞), HT-7 (Shenmen 神门), P-6 (Neiguan 内关), BL-20 (Pishu 脾俞), REN-6 (Qihai 气海)

2. Plegm and Fire Disturbance

ST-40 (Fenglong 丰隆), GB-34 (Yanglingquan 阳陵泉), Ht-4 (Lingdao 灵道), BL-13 (Feishu 肺俞), LU-5 (Chize 尺泽), P-4(Ximen 郄门)

3. Blood Status
HT-3 (Shaohai 少海), BL-17 (Geshu 膈俞), REN-6 (Qihai 气海), P-6 (Neiguan 内关), P-3 (Quze 曲泽)

- **Remarks**
Palpitation is cardiac condition characterized by rapid heartbeat with nervousness and anxiety which may be symptoms in neurosis, functional disorders of nervous system and cardiac arrhythmia.

1-25 Retention of Urine 癃闭 Longbi

- **Differentiation**

1. Accumulation of Damp-Heat in the Urinary Bladder
The manifestations are distention in the lower abdomen, hot scanty urine, thirst but no desire to drink, red tongue with yellow coating, rapid pulse.

2. Kidney-Qi Deficient
The manifestations are dribbling of urine, lumbar soreness, listlessness, pallor complexion, weakness of knee, pale tongue, deep thready pulse.

3. Urethral Obstruction
The manifestations are dribbling of urine, pain and distention in lower abdomen, red spot on the tongue, rapid pulse.

- **Treatment**
  Prescription
1. Accumulation of Damp-Heat in the Urinary Bladder
   SP-6 (Sanyinjiao 三阴交), SP-9 (Yinlingquan 阴陵泉),
   REN-3 (Zhongji 中极), BL-28 (Pangguangshu 膀胱俞)

2. Kidney-qi Deficient
   BL-23 (Shenshu 肾俞), SP-6 (Sanyinjiao 三阴交), BL-22
   (Sanjiaoshu 三焦俞), REN-6 (Qihai 气海), KI-10 (Yingu 阴
   谷), BL-39 (Weiyang 委阳)

3. Uretharal Obstruction
   REN-3 (Zhonji 中极), SP-6 (Sanyinjiao 三阴交), BL-28
   (Pangguangshu 膀胱俞), ST-28 (Shuidao 水道), KI-5
   (Shuiquan 水泉)

- **Remarks**
  The Kidney deficiency causes the dysfunction of the
  Urinary Bladder which controls urination.

1-26 Rheumatoid Arthritis 类风湿关节炎
Reifengshiguanjieyan

This is a kind of chronic and immune.
- **Differentiation**
  The manifestations are swelling, stiffness, deformity of
  the joints, pain. It involves wrist, elbow, knee shoulder,
  ankle.
1. Cold-Damp

2. Damp-Heat

- **Treatment**
  Prescription
  ST-36 (Zusanli 足三里), DU-14 (Dazhui 大椎)

1. Upper limbs:
   LI-15 (Jianyu 肩髃), LI-10 (Shousanli 手三里), LI-11 (Quchi 曲池), SJ-15 (Waiguan 外关), LI-4 (Hegu 合谷), Li-5(Yangxi 阳溪), SI-4 (Wangu 腕骨), EX-UE9 (Baxie 八邪)
2. Lower limbs:
   GB-30 (Huantiao 环跳), GB-29 (Juliao 巨髎), EX-LE4 (Xiyan 膝眼), GB-34 (Yanglingquan 阳陵泉), ST-34 (Liangqiu 梁丘), GB-39 (Xuanzhong 悬钟), LIV-8 (Ququan 曲泉), BL-60 (Kunlun 昆仑), ST-41 (Jiexi 解溪), GB-20 (Fengchi 凤池)

(1) Pain:
    GB-20 (Fengchi 凤池), SP-10 (Xuehai 血海), BL-17 (Geshu 膈俞)
(2) Limbs heaviness:
    LI-4 (Hegu 合谷), LI-11 (Quchi 曲池), SP-9 (Sanyinjiao 三阴 交)

Remarks
Moxibution and Ear acupuncture is helpful for curing.

1-27 Seminal Emission 遗精 Yijing

- **Differentiation**

1. Nocturnal Emission
It may be with dreams,
dizziness, palpitation, listlessness, lassitude, yellow urine, red tongue, thready rapid pulse.

2. Involuntary Emission
Frequent mission, pallor complexion, listlessness, soreness in the lumbar region, emaciation, pale tongue, deep thready pulse.

- **Treatment**
Prescription

1. Nocturnal Emission
HT-7 (Shenmen 神门), BL-15 (Xinshu 心俞), BL-23 (Shenshu 肾俞), BL-52 (Zhishi 志室), KI-3 (Taixi 太溪), Ren-4 (Guanyuan 关元), P-6 (Neiguan 内关), SP-6 (Sanyinjiao 三阴交)

2. Involuntary Emission
ST-36 (Zusanli 足三里), BL-23 (Shenshu 肾俞), KI-3 (Taixi 太溪), SP-6 (Sanyinjiao 三阴交), REN-6 (Qihai 气海), REN-4 (Guanyua 关元), KI-12 (Dahe 大赫)

1-28 Schizophrenia 精神分裂症 Jingshenfenliezheng

- **Differentiation**
1. Heart and Liver Fire Exuberance

Excitation, mania, not sleep whole night, glowering eyes, increasing the strength, yellow and brown urine, yellow tongue, and rapid pulse.

2. Phlegm and Qi Stagnation
Mental depression, dull eyes, anorexia, white greasy tongue, slippery pulse.

3. Qi Stagnation and Blood Stasis
Long-term mania, mental instability, delusion, insomnia, dull complexion, dry skin, purplish tongue, and deep pulse.

4. Heat and Spleen Asthenia
Depression, palpitation, palpitation, frighten, inactivity, light coloured tongue, and soft and weak pulse.

- **Treatment**
Prescription
DU-20 (Baihui 百会), P-7 (Daling 大陵), ST-40 (Fenglong 丰隆)
DU-26 (Shuigou 水沟), LU-11 (Shaoshang 少商), P-8 (Laogong 劳宫), DU-14 (Dazhui 大椎), SP-1 (Yinbai 隐白), HT-7 (Shenmen 神门), P-5 (Jianshi 间使), REN-17 (Shanzhong 膻中), LI-4 (Hegu 合谷), LI-11 (Quchi 曲池), LIV-3 (Taichong 太冲), BL-15 (Xinshu 心俞), BL-20 (Pishu 脾俞), ST-36 (Zusanli 足三里), SP-6 (Sanyinjiao 三阴交)

- **Electro acupuncture**
The above prescription points.

1-29 Vomiting 呕吐 Outu

- **Differentiation**
1. Retention of Food
   This is characterized by epigastric distention, casting up of sour tastes, belching, abdominal pain, foul gas, constipation, greasy tongue coating, slippery pulse.

2. Invasion of Stomach by Liver Qi
   This is characterized by vomiting, acid regurgitation, frequent belching, distention in the hypochondriac region, thin greasy tongue coating, wiry pulse.

3. Weakness of Stomach and Spleen
   Sallow complexion, lack of appetite, loose stools, pale, sticky tongue, weak soft pulse.

- **Treatment**
  Prescription
1. Retention of Food
   ST-36 (Zusanli 足三里), P-6 (Neiguan 内关), REN-12 (Zhongwan 中脘), REN-10 (Xiawan 下脘), REN-21 (Xuanji 璇玑), SP-14 (Fujie 腹結)

2. Invation of Stomach by Liver Qi
   ST-36 (Zusanli 足三里), Liv-3 (Taichong 太冲), P-6 (Neiguan 内关), REN-13 (Shangwan 上脘), ST-21 (Liangmen 梁门), GB-34 (Yanglingquan 阳陵泉)

3. Weakness of Stomach and Spleen

BL-20 (Pishu 脾俞), BL.21 (Weishu 胃俞), ST-36 (Zusanli 足三里), SP-4 (Gongsun 公孙), P-6 (Neiguan 内关), SP-9 (Yinlingquan 阴陵泉)

1-30 Windstroke 中风 Zhongfeng

- **Differentiation**

1. Severe Type Attacking the Zangfu

   This condition is critical with sudden onset. The manifestation involves sudden falling down, confused mental state, running saliva from the mouth corner.

(1) Tense Type

   The manifestations are sudden collapse, coma locked jaws, clenched fists and jaws, coarse breathing, grey dark tongue coating, wiry rolling pulse.

(2) Flaccid Type

   The manifestations are sudden falling down, coma, eyes closed, opening mouth, sweat over head and face, incontinence of urine and stools, flaccid tongue, weak thready pulse.

2. Mild Type (Attacking the Channels and Collaterals)

   The condition is mild type. The manifestations are hemiplegia, numbness of skin and limbs, deviation of mouth and eyes, dizziness, yellow greasy tongue coating, wiry slow pulse.

- **Treatment**

Prescription
(Points according to symptoms and signs)
1. Severe Type Attacking the Zangfu
(1) Tense Type
DU-20 (Baihui 百会), KI-1 (Yongquan 涌泉), LIV-3 (Taichong 太冲), ST-40 (Fenglong 丰隆), P-8 (Laogong 劳宫), DU-26 (Shuigou 水沟, Renzhong 人中)
*12 Jing-Well points of both hands

- Clenched jaws: ST-6 (Jiache 颊车), ST-7 (Xiaguan 下关), LI-4 (Hegu 合谷)

- Gurgling with sputum: ST-40 (Fenglong 丰隆), REN-22 (Tiantu 天突)

- Aphasia and stiffness of tongue: Ren-23 (Lianquan 廉泉), DU-15 (Yamen 亚门), HT-5 (Tongli 通里)

(2) Flaccid Type
REN-6 (Qihai 气海), REN-4 (Guanyuan 关元), ST-36 (Zusanli 足三里), DU-26 (Shuigou 水沟, Renzhong 人中)

- Hemiplegia:
DU-20 (Baihui 百会), DU-16 (Fengfu 风府)

- Upper extremity:
LI-11 (Quchi 曲池), SJ-5 (Waiguan 外关), LI-4 (Hegu 合谷), LI-15 (Jianyu 肩髃), GB-34 (Yanglingquan 阳梁泉), ST-36 (Zusanli 足三里), ST-41 (Jiexi 解溪)

2. Mild Type (Attacking the channels and Collaterals)

DU-20 (Baihui 百会), DU-16 (Fengfu 风府), ST-9 (Renying 人迎)

- **Remarks**
  It may be applied in Scalp Acupuncture using motor area and speech area.

- **12 Jing-Well points:**
  LU-11 (Shaoshang 少商), SP-1 (Yinbai 隐白), HT-9 (Shaochong 少冲), KI-1 (Yongquan 涌泉), P-9 (Zhongchong 中冲), LIV-1 (Dadun 大敦), LI-1 (Shangyang 商阳), ST-45 (Lidui 历兑), SI-1, (Shaoze 少泽), BL-67 (Zhiyin 至阴), SJ-1 (Guanchong 关冲), GB-44 (Zuqiaoyin 足窍阴)

- **Scalp acupuncture**
  Motor area, Speech area.

1-31 Wei Syndrome 痿症 Weizheng

- **Differentiation**
  Wei syndrome is characterized by muscular flaccidity or atrophy of the extremities with motor impairment.

1. Heat in the Lung
   It usually occurs during or after a febrile disease. Manifestations are fever, cough, restlessness, thirsty, scanty urine, red tongue with yellow coating, thready rapid pulse.

2. Damp-Heat

The manifestations are heavy sensation of the body, sallow complexion, listlessness, cloudy urine, profuse sweating, hot sensation in the soles of the feet, yellow greasy tongue coating, soft rapid pulse.

3. Liver and Kidney Deficiency
The manifestations are soreness and weakness of the lumbar region, blurring of vision.

4. Trauma
Contusion causes injury of the meridians and leads to retarded Qi and Blood circulation. As a result, the muscles and tendons are poorly nourished, thin white tongue coating, slow hesitant pulse.

- **Treatment**
Prescription
1. Heat in the Lung

- Upper limb:
LI-15 (Jianyu 肩髃), LI-11 (Quchi 曲池), SJ-5 (Waiguan 外关), LI-4 (Hegu 合谷)

- Lower limb:
ST-36 (Zusanli 足三里), ST-31 (Biguan 髀关), ST-41 (Jiexi 解溪), GB-30 (Huantiao 环跳), GB-34 (Yanglingquan 阳陵泉) GB-39 (Xuanzhong 悬钟)

2. Damp-Heat
BL-20 (Pishu 脾俞), SP-9 (Yinlingquan 阴陵泉)

3. Liver and Kidney Deficiency

BL-18 (Ganshu 肝俞), BL-23 (Shenshu 肾俞), KI-3 (Taixi 太溪)

4. Trauma
EX-B2 (Jiaji 夹脊) for spinal injury.

- **Remarks**
It is seen acute myelitis, progressive myatrophy, myasthenia gravis, periodic paralysis and hysterical paralysis.

- **Plum-blossom needle**
Points of hand and foot Yangming meridians, EX-B2 (Jiaji 夹脊)

B2. Gynecology

2-1 Amenorrhea 闭经 Bijing

- **Differentiation**

1.Blood Stasis
This type of Amenorrhea is characterized by an absence of menses, distention and pain in the lower abdomen, aggravated by pressing, but relieved by warmth, purplish dark tongue, deep wiry pulse.

2. Blood Deficiency
This type of Amenorrhea is characterized by delayed menstrual period, and gradually decreasing in amount of flow. It is accompanied by soreness in the lumbar

region and knees, dizziness, loose stool, palpitation, pale, white coating tongue, thready, weak pulse.

- **Treatment**

Prescription
1. Blood Stasis

REN-3 (Zhongji 中极), LI-4 (Hegu 合谷), BL-18 (Ganshu 肝俞), BL-19 (Danshu 胆俞), LIV-2 (Xingjian 行间), LIV-3 (Taichong 太冲), SP-6 (Sanyinjiao 三阴交), SP-10 (Xuehai 血海)

2. Blood Deficiency

REN-4 (Guanyuan 关元), REN-6 (Qihai 气海), BL-23 (Shenshu 肾俞), BL-18 (Ganshu 肝俞), BL-20 (Pishu 脾俞), ST-36 (Zusanli 足三里), SP-6 (Sanyinjiao 三阴交)

- **Remarks**

This refers to female who does not have an experience to get menstrual flow at the age of 18, and also female who ceased to have menstrual flow over three months.

2-2 Dysmenorrhea 痛经 Tongjing

- **Differentiation**

1. Status of Qi and Blood

This type is premenstrual cramping pain fixed in the lower abdomen.

Distending pain of lower abdomen with distention in the breast and the hypochondriac region which appears before or after menstrual flow, accompanied by dripping of scanty dark purplish in colour with clots, dark purplish tongue, wiry pulse.

2. Liver and Kidney Yin Deficiency

This type of lower abdominal pain at late stage of menstruation or post menstruation, and relieved by pressing during or post the menstrual flow. It is mild pain but persistent pain. The scanty flow and pink in colour, may be accompanied by dizziness, palpitation, soreness in the lumbar region and knees, thin white tongue coating, deep thready pulse.

- **Treatment**

  Prescription

1. Status of Qi and Blood

   SP-10 (Xuehai 血海), LI-4 (Hegu 合谷), SP-6 (Sanyinjiao 三阴交), LIV-3 (Taichong 太冲)

2. Liver and Kidney Yin Deficiency

   REN-4 (Guanyuan 关元), BL-20 (Pishu 脾俞), BL-23 (Senshu 肾俞), ST-36 (Zusanli 足三里), SP-6 (Sanyinjiao 三阴交), BL-18 (Ganshu 肝俞)

- **Remarks**

It refers to the periodic pain, and in severe case, it may be involved the lower abdomen, affecting the lumbosacral region.

2-3 Irregular Menstruation 月经不调 Yuejingbutiao

- **Differentiation**

1. Precede Menstrual Flow
   The flow is advanced at least more than seven days, and it may appear fresh red or purple red colour. The symptoms appear irritability, dry mouth, night sweating, feverish palms and soles, red tongue with less coating, rapid thready pulse.

2. Delayed Menstrual Flow
   This condition may the type of deficiency or excess factors. Deficiency caused by deficiency nutrient blood or Yang Qi. Excess caused by stagnation of Qi and Blood of Chong and Ren Channels, which leads to delayed menstrual flow.

3. Disorder of Menstrual Flow
   This condition is mostly caused by impaired circulation of Qi and Blood due to stagnation of Liver Qi, deficiency of Kidney Qi, and the factors are such as emotional depression, anger, as a result, it become disorderly menstrual flow.

- **Treatment**
  Prescription

1. Precede Menstrual Flow
   REN-6 (Qihai 气海), SP-6 (Sanyinjiao 三阴交), SP-1 (Yinbai 隐白), ST-36 (Zusanli 足三里)

2. Delayed Menstrual Flow
   SP-6 (Sanyinjiao 三阴交), SP-8 (Diji 地机), LI-4 (Hegu 合谷), BL-17 (Geshu 膈俞), REN-4 (Guanyua 关元)

3. Disorder of Menstrual Flow
   LIV-3 (Taichong 太冲), SP-6 (Sanyinjiao 三阴交), BL-18 (Ganshu 肝俞), REN-3 (Zhongji 中极)

- **Remarks**
  It refers to cycle, duration, colour, quantity. These are related to environmental change and emotional disturbance.

2-4 Infertility 不孕症 Buyunzheng

- **Differentiation**
1. Kidney Deficiency
   It relates to irregular menstruations, and scanty flow of light red colour. The manifestations are tinnitus, dizziness, soreness of lumbar region and knee, pale white tongue coating, and deep thready pulse.

2. Blood Deficiency
   It relates to scanty flow light red colour, and delayed menstruation. The manifestations are emaciation, dizziness, lassitude, pale tongue with little coating, deep thready pulse.

3. Cold in Uterus
   It relates to have normal menstruation, but its cycle is sometimes prolonged with dark clots. The manifestations are cold limbs, pain in the lower abdomen, profuse urine, pale tongue with white coating, and deep slow pulse.

4. Phlegm-Damp Retention
   It relates an obese constitution, prolonged cycle, profuse sticky leukorrhea, dizziness, palpitation, white sticky tongue coating, and soft slippery pulse.

- **Treatment**
  Prescription
1. Kidney Deficiency
   DU-4 (Mingmen 命门), BL-23 (Shenshu 肾俞), SP-6 (Sanyinjiao 三阴交), KI-3 (Taixi 太溪)

2. Blood Deficiency
   SP-6 (Sanyinjiao 三阴交), REN-6 (Qihai 气海), ST-36 (Zusanli 足三里), EX-CA1 (Zigong 子宫)

3. Cold in Uterus
   DU-4 (Mingmen 命门), REN-4 (Guanyuan 关元), EX-CA1 (Zigong 子宫), Moxibution

4. Phlegm-Damp Retention
   REN-3 (Zhongji 中极), SP-6 (Sanyinjiao 三阴交), SP-8 (Diji 地极), ST-30 (Qichong 气冲), ST-40 (Fenlong 丰隆)

2-5 Lactation Deficiency 乳汁少 **Ruzhishao**

- **Differentiation**

1. Qi and Blood Deficiency
   It is characterized by scanty or absence of milk after childbirth or decrease in quantity during lactation. The breasts feel soft with no distention. The manifestations are loose stools, lassitude, anorexia, pale tongue with less coating, and weak thready pulse.

2. Liver Qi Stagnation
   There is insufficiency or absence of milk production, and appear anorexia, hypochondriac pain, fullness in chest, emotional depression, irritability, thin yellow tongue, wiry, rapid pulse.

- **Treatment**
   Prescription
1. Qi and Blood Deficiency
   ST-18 (Rugen 乳根), SI-1 (Shaoze 少泽), REN-17 (Shanzhong 膻中), BL-20 (Pishu 脾俞, ST-36 (Zusanli 足三里)

2. Liver Qi Stagnation
   P-6 (Neiguan 内关), LIV-14 (Qimen 气门), ST-18 (Rugen 乳根), REN-17(Shanzhong 膻中), SI-1 (Shaozeshao 少泽)

- **Remarks**
   In TCM, milk is transformed from Qi and Blood.

2-6 Leukorrhea 带下 **Daixia**

- **Differentiation**
  Leukorrhea may be differentiated as white or yellow discharge.

1. Spleen Deficiency
   White or slight yellowish of sticky quality without foul smell. The manifestations are loose stool, sallow complexion, lassitude, pale tongue with sticky coating, and slow weak pulse.

2. Kidney Deficiency
   It may be much white and dilute quality discharge, accompanied by soreness in the lumbar region, loose stool, frequent urination, pale tongue with white coating, and deep slow pulse.

3. Damp-Heat Retention
   It is Yellow discharge with bad odor, and accompanied by itching in the virgina, scanty urination, thirst, sticky yellow tongue, and rapid slippery pulse.

- **Treatment**
  Prescription
1. Spleen Deficiency
   GB-26 (Daimai 带脉), SP-6 (Sanyinjiao 三阴交), REN-6 (Qihai 气海), BL-30 (Baihuanshu 白环俞)

2. Kidney Deficiency

GB-26 (Daimai 带脉), SP-6 (Sanyinjiao 三阴交), REN-6 (Qihai 气海), REN-4 (Guanyuan 关元), BL-23 (Senshu 肾俞), KI-6 (Zhaohai 照海), ST-36 (Zusanli 足三里)

3. Damp-Heat Retention
   GB-26 (Daimai 带脉), SP-6 (Sanyinjiao 三阴交), REN-6 (Qihai 气海), SP-9 (Yinlingquan 阴陵泉), LIV-2 (Xingjian 行间), GB-39 (Xuanzhong 悬钟), BL-32 (Ciliao 次髎), REN-3 (Zhonji 中极)

- **Remarks**
  It refers to white discharge of an abnormal colour, quality and odor.

2-7 Morning Sickness 孕吐 Yuntu

- **Differentiation**

1. Spleen and Stomach Deficiency
   It is characterized by distention in the hypochondriac region with nausea, vomiting ma take place right after food intake or smell of food. The symptoms are accompanied with dizziness, lassitude, shortness of breath, palpitation, pale tong with white sticky coating, and slow slippery pulse.

2. Liver and Stomach Incoordination
   It is characterized by vomiting of bitter or sour fluid. They symptoms are fullness in the chest, pain the hypochondriac region, belching, dizziness, excessive

thirst, bitter taste in the mouth, pale tongue, and wiry slippery pulse.

- **Treatment**
Prescription
1. Spleen and Stomach Deficiency
ST-36 (Zusanli 足三里), P-6 (Neiguan 内关), REN-12 (Zhongwan 中脘), SP-4 (Gongsun 公孙) , BL-21 (Weishu 胃俞)

2. Liver and Stomach Incoordination
REN-12 (Zhongwan 中脘), ST-36 (Zusanli 足三里) LIV-3 (Taichong 太冲), P-6 (Neiguan 内关)

- **Remarks**
Morning sickness which is pregnant obstruction, such as vomiting. It is the early reaction of pregnancy during the first three months.

2-8 Malposition of Fetus 胎位不正 Taiweibuzheng

- **Differentiation**
Malposition of Fetus means that the fetus is in an abnormal position in the uterus after thirty weeks of pregnancy. It is often seen in multipara or pregnant women who have laxity of the abdominal wall.

- **Treatment**

BL-67 (Zhiyi 至阴) with Moxibution for 15 minutes for 1-2 times every day until the position of the fetus is normal.

- **Remarks**

Treatment for sitting position on the chair or lies down. According to the history of report shows 80 % of the rate of success.

2-9 Metrorrhagia 出血性 Chuxiexing

- **Differentiation**
1. Spleen Deficiency

   Sudden profuse metrorrhagia is scanty bleeding in light red colour, lassitude, shortness of breath, poor appetite, loose stool, pale tongue with thin white coating, and weak thready pulse.

2. Kidney Deficiency

   The symptoms include profuse of dripping bleeding of light red colour, cold limbs, soreness in the lower back and knees, pale tongue with white coating, and deep thready pulse.

3. Blood Heat Retention

   The manifestations are deep red colour, restlessness, thirst, constipation, red tongue with yellow greasy coating, and rapid full pulse.

- **Treatment**

Prescription

REN-4 (Guanyuan 关元), SP-1 (Yinbai 隐白), SP-6 (Sanyinjiao 三阴交)

- Spleen Deficiency: ST-36 (Zusanli 足三里), BL-20 (Pishu 脾俞)
- Kidney Deficiency: KI-3 (Taixi 太溪)
- Heat in Blood: SP-10 (Xuehai 血海), LIV-2 (Xingjian 行间)

- **Remarks**
  Metrorrhagia refers to the uterine type that bleeds irrelevant to the normal menses.

2-10 Menopause 绝经 Juejing

It is usually seen in woman who is about 55 years old, and at the period before or after termination.

- **Manifestation**
  The manifestations are sudden termination or disorder of menstruation, and flushed face, lassitude, sweating, listlessness, depression, irritability, insomnia, palpitation.

- **Treatment**
  ST-36 (Zusanli 足三里), SP-6 (Sanyinjiao 三阴交), LIV-3 (Taichong 太冲), P-6 (Neiguan 内关), HT-5 (Tongli 通里)

C3. Surgical and Dermatological Disease

3-1 Acne 痤疮 Cuochuang

- **Differentiation**

  Acne is most cases on face, which may release white bodies upon squeezing. This follows by the formation of small pustules with tidal feverish, itching and pain sensation.

- **Treatment**

  Prescription

  SP-6 (Sanyinjiao 三阴交), LIV-3 (taichong 太冲), LI-4 (Hegu 合谷), LI-11 (Quchi 曲池), GB-20 (Fengchi 凤池), BL-13 (Feishu 肺俞), DU-10 (Lingtai 灵台)

- **Remarks**

  Acne is mostly caused by Heat in the skin such as Wind-Heat and retention of Heat.

3-2 Eczema 湿疹 Shizhen

- **Differentiation**

1. Acute

   It is characterized by a rapid onset of erythema. The clusters and flakes may break by scratching, and it may turn into severe itching sensation, red tongue with sticky coating, and rapid slippery pulse.
2. Chronic

After repeated attacking eczema for a long time, it may be caused blood deficiency. The manifestations are roughness of skin, red tongue with less coating, and rapid thready pulse.

- **Treatment**

  Prescription
  1. Acute
     DU-14 (Dazhui 大椎), LI-11 (Quchi 气海), SP-6 (Sanyinjiao 三阴交), SP-9 (Yinlingquan 阴陵泉), DU-10 (Lingtai 灵台)

  2. Chronic
     SP-6 (Sanyinjiao 三阴交), SP-10 (Xuehai 血海), ST-36 (Zusanli 足三里), LIV-3 (Taichong 太冲), BL-17 (Geshu 膈俞), DU-10 (Lingtai 灵台)

3-3 Goiter 甲状腺肿 Jiazhuangxianzhong/Qiying 气瘿

Goiter is characterized to an enlargement of thyroid gland, causing a swelling in the front part of the neck.

- **Differentiation**
  Swelling of the neck, which may be accompanied by stuffiness in the chest, palpitation, shortness of breath, wiry, rolling pulse.

- **Treatment**
  Prescription

REN-22 (Tiantu 天突), SJ-17 (Yifeng 翳风), LI-4 (Hegu 合谷), ST-40 (Fenglong 丰隆), ST-36 (Zusanli 足三里), LI-17 (Tianding 天鼎), SI-17 (Tianrong 天容), SJ-13 (Naohui 臑会)

- **Remarks**
  It may be caused by anxiety or mental depression which leads to stagnation of Qi and accumulate fluid forming phlegm.

3-4 Herpes Zoster 带状疱疹
Daizhuangpaozhen/Chanyaohuodan

It is known as heat rash and it mostly affects the lumbar region.

- **Differentiation**

It occurs mainly small vesicles such as beads forming mostly in the lumbar region and the waist with red coloured blisters. The manifestations are burning pain sensation.

- **Treatment**
  Prescription
  LI-11 (Quchi 曲池), SP-10 (Xuehai 血海), BL-40 (Weizhong 委中), EX-B2 (Jiaji 夹脊), GB-34 (Yanglingquan 阳陵泉)

Addition: according type

1. Wind-Heat type
   LIV-2 (Xingjian 行间), LIV-3 (Taichong 太冲), GB-44 (Zuqiaoyin 足窍阴), GB-41 (Zulinqi 足临泣), DU-10 (Lingtai 灵台), SJ-6 (Zhigou 支沟)

2. Damp-Heat type
   SP-4 (Gongsun 公孙), SJ-5 (Waiguan 外关), ST-44 (Neiting 内庭), ST-36 (Zusanli 足三里), GB-43 (Xiaxi 侠溪)

3-5 Hernia 疝 Shan

- **Differentiation**

  The manifestations are pain of the testis, lower abdomen, swelling and dragging sensation of the scrotum.
  1. Cold Hernia
  2. Damp-Heat Hernia

- **Treatment**
  Prescription
  LIV-3 (Taichong 太冲), REN-3 (Zhongji 中极), REN-4 (Guanyuan 关元), SP-6 (Sanyinjiao 三阴交)

(1) Upper point and Lower point
    ST-36 (Zusanli 足三里), LI-11 (Quchi 曲池), SP-12 (Chongmen 冲门), SP-6 (Sanyinjiao 三阴交)

(2) Liver point

    REN-6 (Qihai 气海), SP-6 (Sanyinjiao 三阴交), KI-3 (Taixi 太溪), LIV-1 (Dadun 大敦)

228

(3) Point Zhishanxue (0.5 cun anterior to KI-6 (Zhaohai 照
海)

- **Remarks**
Moxibution: point LIV-1 (Dadun 大敦), SJ-4 (Yangchi 阳
池), M-CA-23 (Sanjiaojiu)Triangular Moxibution.

3-6 Hemorrhoids 痔疮 Zhichuang

It refers to swollen or small pieces of muscle exposed on
the anus internally or externally.

- **Differentiation**

1.Internal Hemorrhoids
Damp-Heat Retention:
It involves pain in the anus, and small soft swollen veins
in fresh red or purplish green colour. The
manifestations are feverish sensation in the anus,
constipation, red tongue, and rapid pulse.
Qi Deficiency:
The manifestation, pallor complexion, shortness of
breath, poor appetite, no energy, prolapse of swollen
veins, pale tongue, and weak thready pulse.
2. External Hemorrhoids
The manifestations are visible swollen veins with big
size and hard in nature. It may be caused by long sitting,
long standing and anus friction which does not involve
bleeding.

- **Treatment**
Prescription

1.Damp-Heat Retention
   LI-4 (Hegu 合谷), LI-11 (Quchi 曲池), LU-6 (Kongzui 孔最), BL-57 (Chengshan 承山), P-4 (Ximen 郄门), EX-UE-2 (Erbai 二白), DU-20 (Baihui 百会), SP-5 (Shangqiu 商丘)

2. Qi Deficiency
   LU-6 (Kongzui 孔最), REN-6 (Qihai 气海), DU-20 (Baihui 百会), BL-57 (Chengshan 承山) , P-4 (Ximen 郄门), BL-30 (Baihuanshu 白环俞)

- **Remarks**
   Moxibution with point DU-20 (Baihui 白会), REN-6 (Qihai 气海).

3-7 Heel Pain 脚跟痛 Jiaogentong

- **Differentiation**

   The manifestations are mainly sprain, pain creating on heel contact with the ground and difficult to walk.

- **Treatment**
   Prescription
   ST-7 (Xiaguan 下关), K-3 (Taixi 太溪), Ashi point.

- **Remarks**
   Alternative: Roll the tennis ball back and forth with the sole of your foot many times.

3-8 Neck Sprain 颈扭伤 Jingniushang

Neck sprain is characterized by difficult turning the neck.

- **Differentiation**

The manifestations are, most patients have limited movement and difficulty to turn to other and back side, and it may be radiate towards shoulder and arm, but no swelling and redness on the skin, thin white tongue, and wiry tense pulse.

- **Treatment**
Prescription
GB-20 (Fengchi 凤池), DU-14 (Dazhui 大椎), SI-3 (Houxi 后溪), SI-14 (Jianwaishu 肩外俞), BL-10 (Tianzhu 天杼), GB-21 (Jianjing 肩井)

3-9 Psoriasis 银屑病 Yinxiebing

It refers to a chronic skin condition characterized by repeated scaled dermatosis, and have some dry silver, white scales covered.

- **Differentiation**

1. Damp-Heat with Wind
   The manifestations are, red tongue with yellow greasy tongue coating, and rapid soft pulse.

2. Blood Deficiency with Dry Wind
   The manifestations are, red tongue with white coating, and thready weak pulse.

- **Treatment**
  Prescription
  1. Damp-Heat with Wind
     Li-4 (Hegu 合谷), LI-11 (Quchi 曲池), GB-20 (Fengchi 凤池), BL-17 (Geshu 膈俞), SP-9 (Yinlingquan 阴陵泉), SP-3 (Taibai 太白), ST-9 (Renying 人迎)

  2. Blood Deficiency with Dry Wind
     LI-4 (Hegu 合谷), LI-11 (Quchi 曲池), SP-6 (Sanyinjiao 三阴交), SP-10 (Xuehai 血海), ST-9 (Renying 人迎), ST-36 (Zusanli 足三里)

3-10 Tennis Elbow

This sometimes happen when sportsman's play racket with rotation of forearm and flexion of elbow joint.

- **Differentiation**

The Manifestations are exposure to cold and wind attack to forearm, pain of the lateral side of the elbow, and it is more painful to extending or rotating of the elbow.

- **Treatment**
  LI-11 (Quchi 曲池), LI-12 (Zhouliao 肘髎), Ashi point, GB 34 (Yanglingquan 阳陵泉)

3-11 Urticaria 荨麻疹 **Xunmazhen**

It is abrupt onset with itching flat-topped wheals of various size on the skin. In TCM, it calls Wind Wheal.

- **Differentiation**

1. Wind Heat
   The manifestations are red rashes, severe itching, rapid pulse.

2. Wind Damp
   The manifestations are Light red or white rashes superficial and rapid pulse.
3. Accumulation of Heat in the Stomach and Intestine
   The manifestations are, red rashes, abdominal pain, constipation, diarrhea, thin yellow tongue coating, and rapid pulse.

- **Treatment**
  Prescription
  SP-6 (Sanyinjiao 三阴交), SP-10 (Xuehai 血海), LI-11 (Quchi 曲池), LI-4 (Hegu 合谷), ST-36 (Zusanli 足三里), BL-40 (Weizhong 委中), SP-9 (Yinlingquan 阴陵泉)

D4. Pediatric Diseases

4-1 Enuresis 遗尿症 **Yiniaozheng**

It refers to involuntary discharge of the urine of a child. It happens to occur during sleep.

- **Differentiation**

It may be happened in several nights during sleep. The manifestations are listlessness, poor appetite.

- **Treatment**
Prescription
REN-3 (Zhongji 中极), REN-4 (Guanyuan 关元), BL-23 (Shenshu 肾俞), SP-6 (Sanyinjiao 三阴交), ST-36 (Zusanli 足三里)

- **Remarks**
Moxibution may be applied.

4-2 Infantile Convulsion 小儿惊风 Xiaoerjingfeng

Infants are not physically developed, and they are mentally weak.

- **Differentiation**

1. Acute Convulsion
The manifestations are high fever, clenched jaws, upward staring eyes, contraction, rattles, rapid and wiry pulse.

2. Chronic Convulsion
The manifestations are pallor, lassitude, emaciation, intermittent convulsion, loose stools, clear urine, weak pulse.

- **Treatment**

  Prescription
  LI-11 (Quchi 曲池), DU-26 (Renzhong 人中, Shuigou 水沟), EX-UE-11 (Shixuan 十宣)
  1. Points for different symptoms and sign

     Protracted Convulsion: LIV-2 (Xingjian 行间), GB-34 (Yanglingquan 阳陵泉), BL-60 (Kunlun 昆仑), SI-3 (Houxi 后溪)

     High Fever: LI-4 (Hegu 合谷), DU-14 (Dazhui 大椎)
     Coma: KI-1 (Yongquan 涌泉), P-8 (Laogong 劳宫)

- **Remarks**
  Point EX-UE-11 (Shixuan 十宣) locates on the tips of the ten fingers, 0.1 cun distal to end of the nails.

4-3 Infantile Diarrhea 小儿腹泻 Xiaoerfuxie

It is a common pediatric disease, mainly manifested by frequent bowel movement, watery feces. It may occur in any season, but more often occurs in summer and autumn.

- **Differentiation**
  1. Cold-Damp

The stool is watery, abdominal pain, accompanied by aversion to cold, pale tongue with thin coating, and thin deep pulse.

2. Damp-Heat

The manifestations are the yellowish stool, watery, feverish sensation, yellow and greasy tongue coating, slippery rapid pulse.

3. Food Retention

The manifestations are epigastric distension that alleviated by bowel movement, poor appetite, vomiting, thick yellow greasy tongue coating, full slippery pulse.

4. Yang Deficiency

It characterized by watery stool, cold limbs, poor spirit, pale tongue with white coating, and thready pulse.

- **Treatment**

  Prescription

  REN-12 (Zhongwan 中脘), ST-25 (Tianshu 天枢), ST-37 (Shangjuxu 上巨虚), EX-UE10 (Sifeng 四缝)

1. Cold-Damp

   REN12 (Zhongwan 中脘), ST-36 (Zusanli 足三里), ST-25 (Tianshu 天枢), REN-8 (Shenque 神阙), REN-4 (Guanyuan 关元)

2. Damp-Heat

   ST-25 (Tianshu 天枢), REN-12 (Zhongwan 中脘), ST-36 (Zusanli 足三里), ST-44 (Neiting 内庭), LI-11 (Quchi 曲池)

3. Food Retention
   REN-12 (Zhongwan 中脘), ST-25 (Tianshu 天枢), ST-36 (Zusanli 足三里), REN-6 (Qihai 气海), ST-44 (Neiting 内庭)

4. Yang Deficiency
   DU-20 (Baihuibaihui 百会), ST-36 (Zusanli 足三里), REN-12 (Zhongwan 中脘), BL-20 (Pishu 脾俞), BL-23 (Shenshu 肾俞), LIV-13 (Zhangmen 章门)

- **Remarks**
  The case of catch cold, add point LI-4 (Hegu 合谷).

4-4 Infantile Paralysis 小儿麻痹 **Xiaoermabi**

It is due to invasion of epidemic pathogenic factors that injure the meridians.

- **Differentiation**

  Paralysis may be the part of body, especially lower limb, and there is muscular atrophy of the affected part with deformity of the trunk.

- **Treatment**
  Prescription
  Upper limb paralysis:
  LI-11 (Quchi 曲池), LI-4 (Hegu 合谷), LI-15 (Jianyu 肩髃), DU-14 (Dazhui 大椎), BL-10 (Tianzhu 天柱), SJ-5 (Waiguan 外关)

  Lower limb paralysis:

ST-36 (Zusanli 足三里), ST-41 (Jiexi 解溪), GB-30 (Huantiao 环跳), GB-34 (Yanglingquan 阳陵泉), GB-39 (Xuanzhong 悬钟), ST-31 (Biguan 髀关), BL-60 (Kunlun 昆仑), SP-6 (Sanyinjiao 三阴交)

dominal muscles paralysis:
ST-25 (Tianshu 天枢), ST-21 (Liangmen 梁门), REN-4 (Guanyuan 关元), GB-26 (Daimai 带脉)

Hand paralysis:
SI-3 (Houxi 后溪), LI-5 (Yangxi 阳溪), SJ-4 (Yangchi 阳池), SJ-9 (Sidu 四读), HT-3 (Shaohai 少海).

4-5 Infantile Fever 小儿发热 Xiaoerfare

- **Differentiation**

It is often caused by attacking of exogenous pathogenic wind, and improper intake of food and milk with retention of food in the interior.
1. Invading Lung and Stomach
2. Affecting Blood by Pathogenic Heat

- **Treatment**
Prescription
LI-4 (Dazhui 大椎), LI-11 (Quchi 曲池), GB-20 (Fengchi 凤池), SJ-1 (Guanchong 关冲)

Vomiting and nausea
Add P-6 (Neiguan 内关)

- **Remarks**
  Add Ear Acupuncture.
- **Ear acupuncture**
  Shenmen, Sympathetic, Lung, Ear apex, Trachea, Tonsil, Throat, Spleen, Large intestine.

E5. Diseases of Eyes, Ears, Nose and Throat

5-1 Cataract 白内障 Baineizhang

This is divided to Congenital and Acquired.
- **Differentiation**

(1) Congenital
(2) Acquired
  This is mainly affecting those over 50 years old and is characterized by chronic disorder in both eyes. It causes deficiency Liver, Kidney, Spleen, Stomach, Yin deficiency and is failure the essence and blood to prevent eye malnourishment.

- **Treatment**

  Prescription
  BL-1 (Jingming 睛明), GB-14 (Yangbai 阳白), GB-20 (Fengchi 凤池), LI-4 (Hegu 合谷), EX-HN7 (Qiuhou 球后), EX-HN5 (Taiyang 太阳), EX-HN14 (Yiming 翳明), LI-14 (Binao 臂臑), GB-1 (Tongziliao 瞳子髎), SJ-17 (Yifeng 翳

风), GB37 (Guangming 光明), ST-36 (Zusanli 足三里), BL-18 (Ganshu 肝俞), BL-23 (Shenshu 肾俞).

- **Remarks**

Ear acupuncture: Eye region, Liver, Kidney, Adrenal Gland, Heart, Sympathetic Nerve.

5-2 Conjunctivitis 结膜炎 Jiemoyan

Congestion, swelling and pain of the eye in acute.

- **Differentiation**

Invasion for exogenous wind-heat.
The manifestations are swelling and pain, burning sensation in the eyelids, and this is caused by excessive fire in the Liver and Gallbladder, bitter taste in the mouth, dizziness, red tongue with yellow coating, and rapid wiry pulse.

- **Treatment**

LIV-2 (Xingjian 行间), LI-4 (Hegu 合谷), LI-11 (Quchi 曲池), EX-HN5 (Taiyang 太阳), DU-23 (Shangxing 上星), GB-20 (Fengchi 凤池), GB-43 (Xiaxi 侠溪), LU-11 (Shaoshang 少商), BL-1 (Jingming 睛明), LIV-3 (Taichong 太冲), GB-37 (Guangming 关明).

- **Remarks**

Ear acupuncture: Ear zone.

5-3 Deafness and Mute 聋哑 Longya

Deafness is the cause of mute and mute is mostly related to a complete loss of hearing.

- **Differentiation**
  These are referred to complete loss of hearing.

- **Treatment**

  Prescription
  GB-8 (Shuaigu 率谷), GB-5 (Xuanlu 悬颅), GB-9 (Tianchong 天冲), GB-2 (Tinghui 听会), SJ-3 (Zhongzhu 中诸), GB-34 (Yanglingquan 阳陵泉), DU-15 (Yamen 哑门), SI-19 (Tinggong 听宫).

- **Remarks**
  Refer to 5-16 Tinnitus and Deafness.

5-4 Epistaxis 鼻衄 Binü

It refers to nasal bleeding.

- **Differentiation**
1. Lung Heat
   The manifestations are dripping blood by dry nose, dry mouth, fever, cough, red tongue with thin white coating, and rapid superficial pulse.

2. Stomach Heat
The manifestations are deep red colour, dry throat, constipation, scanty urine, red tongue with yellow coating, and rapid superficial pulse.

3. Liver and Kidney Yin Deficiency
The manifestations are dry nose, feverish sensation, cough, red tongue with thin white coating, and rapid superficial pulse.

- **Treatment**

  Prescription
1. Lung Heat
   LI-4 (Hegu 合谷), LU-11 (Shaoshang 少阳), LI-20 (Yingxiang 迎香), GB-20 (Fengchi 凤池)

2. Stomach Heat
   LI-4 (Hegu 合谷), LI-20 (Yingxiang 迎香), DU-23 (Shangxing 上星), ST-45 (Lidui 厉兑), ST-44 (Neiting 内庭)

3. Liver and Kidney Yin Deficiency
   KI-3 (Taixi 太溪), LIV-3 (Taichong 太冲), BL-7 (Tongtian 通天), BL-58 (Feiyang 飞扬)

- **Remarks**
  Epistaxis refers to nasal bleeding caused by traumatic injuries.

5-5 Glaucoma 青光眼 Qingguangyan

It is caused by an emotion which led to fire in the Liver and Gallbladder flaring up the eyes which the fluid could not work properly.

- **Differentiation**

  The manifestations are headache, distention of the eyes, vomiting, congested conjunctiva, cloudiness, and eventually increased optic atrophy, and blindness.

  1. Primary Glaucoma type
  2. Secondary Glaucoma type

- **Treatment**

  Prescription
  LI-4 (Hegu 合谷), LIV-3 (Taichong 太冲), BL-2 (Zanzhu 攒竹), BL-19 (Danshu 胆俞), BL-17 (Geshu 膈俞), BL-23 (Shenshu 肾俞), GB-20 (Fengchi 凤池), KI-3 (Taixi 太溪), SP-6 (Sanyinjiao 三阴交), BL-18 (Ganshu 肝俞)

- **Remarks**
  Ear acupuncture: Eye zone, Liver, Heart, Ear Apex, Hypertensive Groove.

5-6 Myopia 近视 Jinshi

It is characterized in that the eyes can see near objects but not distant.
- **Differentiation**

It is clear for near objects but blurred vision for distant which may be accompanied by tinnitus, insomnia, dizziness, pale tongue, and weak thready pulse.

- **Treatment**

GB1 (Jingming 睛明), ST-1 (Chengqi 承泣), GB-20 (Fengchi 凤池), GB-37 (Guangming 光明), BL-18 (Ganshu 肝俞), BL-23 (Shenshu 肾俞)

- **Remarks**
Ear Acupuncture: Eye zone plus Liver, Kidney Sympathetic point.

5-7 Ottis Media 中耳炎 Zhongeryan

It is characterized by pain in the ear and discharge of purulent substance from the ear.

- **Differentiation**

1. Pathogenic Wind-Heat Invasion
The manifestations are fever, headache, and foul smell will flow out from the ear, red tongue with yellow coating, and rapid and wiry pulse.

2. Retention of Damp
There is a foul smell flows, dizziness, tinnitus, pale tongue with white coating, and weak, thready pulse.

- **Treatment**

244

1. Pathogenic Wind-Heat Invasion
    LI-4 (Hegu 合谷), LIV-2 (Xingjian 行间), GB-20 (Fengchi 凤池), GB-12 (Wangu 完骨), SJ-1 (Guanchong 关冲), Ear apex

2. Retention of Damp
    ST-36 (Zusanli 足三里), SP-9 (Yinlingquan 阴陵泉), SJ-17 (Yifeng 翳风), SP-1 (Yinbai 隐白)

- **Remarks**
  Ear acupuncture: Ear apex, Kidney, Occiput, Outer ear.

5-8 Optic Atrophy 视神经萎缩 Shishenjingweisuo

This is a chronic eye disorder by gradual degeneration of vision.

- **Differentiation**
1. Liver and Kidney Deficiency
    The manifestations are dizziness, tinnitus, dryness of the eye, blurred vision, lower back pain, red tongue with scanty coating, weak pulse.

2. Qi and Blood Deficiency
    The manifestations are lassitude, loose stools, blurred vision, weakness of breath, pale tongue with thin coating, weak thready pulse.

- **Treatment**
  Prescription
  GB-20 (Fengchi 风池), BL-1 (Jingming 睛明), GB-37 (Guangming 光明), EX、HN7 (Qiuhou 球后)
1. Liver and Kidney Deficiency

BL-23 (Shenshu 肾俞), BL-18 (Ganshu 肝俞), LIV-3 (Taicong 太冲), KI-3 (Taixi 太溪)

2. Qi and Blood Deficiency
SP-6 (Sanyinjiao 三阴交), ST-36 (Zusanli 足三里), LIV-14 (Qimen 期门), LIV-3 (Taichong 太冲), GB-34 (Yanlingquan 阳陵泉)

5-9 Rhinitis 鼻炎 Biyan

This is by nasal obstruction and nasal secretion.

- **Differentiation**

  This is induced by the exogenous Wind-Cold or Wind-Heat, improper diet, and the manifestations are nasal secretion of thick and yellow mucosa.

- **Treatment**

  Li-4 (Hegu 合谷), LI-11 (Quchi 曲池), LI-20 (Yingxiang 迎香), DU-14 (Dazhui 大椎), DU-23 (Shangxing 上星), DU-25 (Suliao 素髎), LU-7 ((Lieque 列缺), BL-7 (Tongtian 通天), SP-6 (Sanyinjiao 三阴交)

- **Remarks**
  Add Ear acupuncture, Nose region (internal, external) Endocrine, Adrenal, Lung.

5-10 Sore Throat 咽喉肿 Yanhouzhongtong

It is similar to tonsillitis.

- **Differentiation**

1. Excess Heat
   This is abrupt onset with fever, headache, pain in the throat, constipation, thirst, red tongue with thin yellow coating, superficial rapid pulse.

2. Deficient Heat
   Gradual onset without fever, dry throat, feverish sensation in palms and soles, red uncoated tongue, and rapid thready pulse.

- **Treatment**
  Prescription

1. Excess Heat
   LU-11 (Shaoshang 少商), LI-4 (Hegu 合谷), ST-44 (Neiting 内庭), SI-17 (Tianrong 天容), GB-20 (Fengchi 凤池), LU-7 (Lieque 列缺)

2. Deficient Heat
   KI-3 (Taixi 太溪), LU-7 (Lieque 列缺), LU-10 (Yuji 鱼际), KI-6 (Zhaohai 照海)

- **Remarks**
  Ear acupuncture: Throat, Lung Tonsil, Helix area 1-6.

5-11 Tinnitus and Deafness 耳鸣 耳聋 Erming Erlong

Tinnitus is characterized by continuous ringing of the ear, and Deafness refers to loss of hearing and low degree of hearing.

- **Differentiation**

1. Excess of Liver and Gallbladder

   Tinnitus: It is continuous ringing in the ear and there is no relieving.
   Deafness: Sudden deafness.
   The manifestations are irritability, heavy sensation of the head, bitter taste in mouth, red tongue with yellow coating rapid wiry pulse.

2. Deficiency of Kidney Essence

   Tinnitus: It is intermittent ringing and it becomes aggravated after stress and strain, but it is alleviated by pressure.
   Deafness: It is gradually intensified deafness.
   The manifestations are dizziness, lassitude, low back pain, insomnia, red tongue with little coating, and weak thready pulse.

- **Treatment**
  Prescription
1. Excess of Liver and Gallbladder
   SJ-17 (Yifeng 翳 风), GB-2 (Tinghui 听 会), SJ-3 (Zhongzhu 中诸), SJ-21 (Ermen 耳门), GB-43 (Xiaxi 侠溪),

LIV-2 (Xingjian 行间), GB-41 (Zulinqi 足临泣), SJ-5 (Waiguan 外关)

2. Deficiency of Kidney Essence
   BL-23 (Shenshu 肾俞), KI-3 (Taixi 太溪), SJ-17 (Yifeng 翳风), SJ-3 (Zhongzhu 中杼), GB-2 (Tinghui 听会), DU-4 (Mingmen 命门), REN-4 (Guanyuan 关元), SP-6 (Sanyinjiao 三阴交).

- **Remarks**
  Scalp acupuncture: Hearing region.

5-12 Toothache 齿痛 Chitong

- **Differentiation**

1. Wind-Heat
   Toothache follows swelling, pain, preference for cold food, fever, constipation, red tongue with white coating, and rapid pulse.

2. Kidney Deficiency
   Toothache follows intermittent pain, loose teeth, red tongue, and rapid thready pulse.

- **Treatment**
  Prescription
1. Wind-Heat
   ST-44 (Neiting 内庭), GB-20 (Fengchi 凤池), LI-4 (Hegu 合谷), ST-6 (Jiache 颊车), ST-7 (Xiaguan 下关)

2. Kidney Deficiency

KI-3 (Taixi 太溪), LI-4 (Hegu 合谷), ST-6 (Jiach 颊车), ST-7 (Xiaguan 下关)

5-13 Trigeminal Neuralgia 三叉神经痛 Sanchashenjingtong (Facial Pain 面部疼痛 Mianbutengtong)

Trigeminal nerves are divided into three branches, which are supraorbital branch, maxillary branch and mandibular branch.

- **Differentiation**

  It is manifested by sudden onset of facial pain, occurs in transient paroxysms, and just like being cutting, burning and needling, which lasts in a few seconds or few minutes, and several times a day. It is accompanied by local spasm, lacrimation and salivation.

- **Treatment**
  Prescription
  (1)   Main points:
         ST-44 (Neiting 内庭), LI-4 (Hegu 合谷), ST-7 (Xiaguan 下关)

  (2)   Then, combine the other points according to different   symptoms and pain location.

ST-2 (Sibai 四白), ST-6 (Jiache 颊车), ST-4 (Dicang 地仓), REN-24 (Chengjian 承浆), GB-14 (Yangbai 阳白), BL-2 (Cuanzhu, zanzhu 攒竹), SJ-3 (Zhongzhu 中诸), GB-41

(Zulinqi 足临泣), LIV-3 (Taichong 太冲), EX-HN5 (Taiyang 太阳), EX-HN4 (Yuyao 鱼腰)

- **Remarks**
Trigeminal Neuralgia is referred to Facial pain.

F6.   Miscellaneous

6-1 Cervical Spondylopathy 颈椎病 Jingchuibing

- **Manifestation**

Pain in the around the neck, forearm, shoulder, movement of the head, numbness in the lower limbs, heavy sensation, dizziness, headache.

- **Treatment**
Prescription
GB-20 (Fengchi 凤池), LI-11 (Quchi 曲池), LI-15 (Jianyu 肩髃), LI-4 (Hegu 合谷), SI-3 (Houxi 后溪), EX-B2 (Jiaji 夹脊), ST-36 (Zusanli 足三里), GB-34 (Yanlingquan 阳陵泉)

- **Alternative treatment**

Plum blossom Needle:
EX-B2 (Jiaji 夹脊)

6-2 Cosmesis 美容 Meirong

Cosmetic acupuncture, which helps to promote Qi and Blood circulation by needling.

- **Treatment**
  Prescription
  1. Wrinkle:
  GB-1 (Tongziliao 瞳子髎), EX-HN5 (Taiyang 太阳), GB-14 (Yangbai 阳白), ST-3 (Juliao 巨髎), ST-2 (Sibai 四白), SI-18 (Quanliao 顴髎), LI-20 (Yingxiang 迎香), BL-1 (Jingming 睛明), LIV-5 (Ligou 蠡沟), LIV-3 (Taichong 太冲), SP-9 (Yinlingquan 阴陵泉), BL-18 (Ganshu 肝俞), BL-20 (Pishu 脾俞), ST-36 (Zusanli 足三里), SI-3 (Houxi 后溪), LI-4 (Hegu 合谷), SJ-6 (Waiguan 外关)

- **Remarks**
  Ear acupuncture: Endocrine, Cheek, Adrenal, Lung, Shenmen.
  Face massage may be increased to help Qi and Blood circulation.

6-3 Facial Paralysis 面瘫 Miantan
Deviation of Eye and Mouth 口眼歪斜 Kouyanwaixi

Deviated mouth and eyes are the common name. The paralysis appears mostly on one side, mostly among young and middle-aged people.

- **Differentiation**

  This is caused by weakness of the channels, which are attacked by the exogenous pathogenic wind-cold or

252

wind-heat and led to the flaccidness of muscles by Qi stagnation and blood stasis in the channels of face.

- **Treatment**
  Prescription
  ST-4 (Dicang 地仓), ST-6 (Jiache 颊车), LIV-3 (Taichong 太冲), LI-4 (Hegu 合谷), EX-HN5 (Taiyang 太阳), GB-14 (Yangbai 阳白), ST-2 (Sibai 四白), ST-7 (Xiaguan 下关), SJ-17 (Yifeng 翳风), SI-18 (Quanliao 颧髎), LI-20 (Yingxiang 迎香)

6-4 Obesity 肥胖 Feipang

It refers to excessive accumulation of fat in the body tissues. Clinically, it is divided into Simple and Secondary types.
Simple Obesity: It is due to overeating of greasy, sweet food that exceeds the normal consumption of body heat.
Secondary Obesity: It is caused by hypothalamic pituitary lesions and over-secretion of hydrocortisone.

- **Manifestations**

Patients have visible fat accumulations in the neck, lower abdomen and buttock. Mild obese patients do not have signs of symptom, but severe patients have metabolic disturbances of aversion to heat, profuse sweating, fatigue, dizziness, headache, palpitation.

- **Treatment**
  prescription

ST-25 (Tianshu 天枢), REN-9 (Shuifen 水分), REN-12 (Zhongwan 中脘), REN-6 (Qihai 气海), REN-4 (Guanyuan 关元), ST-28 (Shuidao 水道), SP-14 (Fujie 腹結), SP-15 (Daheng 大横), GB-26 (Daimai 带脉), LI-4 (Hegu 合谷), LI-11 (Quchi 曲池), SJ-6 (Zhigou 支沟), SP-10 (Xuehai 血海), SP-11 (Jimen 簋门), ST-32 (Futu 伏兔), SP-6 (Sanyinjiao 三阴交), ST-36 (Zusanli 足三里), ST-44 (Neiting 内庭)

- **Remarks**

Ear acupuncture can be used at the same time as body acupuncture.

6-5 Stopping Smoking 戒烟 Jieyan

It means eliminating addiction to smoking cigarettes. In TCM, smoking affects the function of Lung, Heart, Pericardium, Spleen, Stomach, and leads to disfunction of Pulmonary Qi.

- **Differentiation**

Symptom: Stopping Smoking may be led to restlessness, discomfort in the throat, yawning, blurred vision, weakness, and inability to work normally.

- **Treatment**

LI-4 (Hegu 合谷), LU-7 (Lieque 列缺), ST-36 (Zusanli 足三里), LU-6 (Kongzui 孔最), HT-7 (Shenmen 神门), SP-6 (Sanyinjiao 三阴交), ST-6 (Jiache 颊车), GB-20 (Fengchi 凤池), DU-20 (Baihui 百会), EX-HN3 (Yintang 印堂)

6-6 Sciatica 坐骨神经 **Zuogushenjingtong**

This is the pain radiating to the sciatic nerve distribution in the hip region, posterior lateral aspect of the leg.

- **Manifestations**

1. Primary Sciatica
   It is characterized by a sudden onset of continuous sharp pain, worsens with cold, alleviates with warmth.

2. Secondary Sciatica
   This is a slow onset of pain which may involve primary lesions, radiating pain due to lumbar disc degeneration. The pain is worse with cough, sneezing.

- **Treatment**
   Prescription
1. Primary Sciatica
   GB-30 (Huantiao 环跳), GB-31 (Fengshi 风市), GB-34 (Yanglingquan 阳陵泉), BL-57 (Chengshan 承山), BL-60 (Kunlun 昆仑)

2. Secondary Sciatica
   GB-34 (Yanglingquan 阳陵泉), GB-39 (Xuanzhong 悬钟), BL-25 (Dachangshu 大肠俞), BL-26 (Guanyuanshu 关元俞), BL-54 (Zhibian 秩边), BL-40 (Weizhong 委中), EX-B2 (Huatuojiaji 夹脊) L4 to L5

6-7 Sprain 扭挫伤 **Niucuoshang**

- **Differentiation**
  The manifestations are local soreness, distension, redness, swelling, and the movement is limited.

- **Treatment**
  Prescription
  Ashi points 啊是穴

(1) Neck: BL-10 (Tianzhu 天柱), SI-3 (Houxi 后溪)
(2) Shoulder: GB-21 (Jianjing 肩井), LI-15 (Jianyu 肩髃)
(3) Elbow: LI-11 (Quchi 曲池), LI-4 (Hegu 合谷)

(4) Wrist: SJ-4 (Yangchi 阳池), SJ-5 (Waiguan 外关)
(5) Hip: GB-30 (Huantiao 环跳), GB-34 (Yanglingquan 阳陵泉)
(6) Knee: ST-35 (Dubi 犊鼻), ST-44 (Neiting 内庭)
(7) Ankle: ST-41 (Jiexi 解溪), GB-40 (Qiuxu 丘墟), BL-60 (Kunlun 昆仑)

CHARPTER 4 Ear Acupuncture Therapy

I. Anatomical Structure of the Auricular Surface

To facilitate location of Ear Points, Anatomical Structures of the Auricular surface relating to Ear Acupuncture are as follows.

1. Helix 耳
2. Helix Tubercle 耳轮结节
3. Helix Cauda 耳轮尾
4. Helix Crus 耳轮脚
5. Antihelix 对耳轮
6. The principal part of Antihelix 对耳轮体
7. Superior Antihelix Crus 对耳轮上脚
8. Inferior Antihelix Crus 对耳轮下脚
9. Triangular Fossa 三角窝
10. Scapha 耳舟
11. Tragus 耳屏
12. Supratragic Notch 屏上切迹
13. Antitragus 对耳屏
14. Intertragic Notch 屏间切迹
15. Helix Notch 轮屏切迹
16. Ear Lobe 耳垂
17. Concha 甲腔
18. Cymba Concha 耳甲艇
19. Cavity Concha 耳甲腔

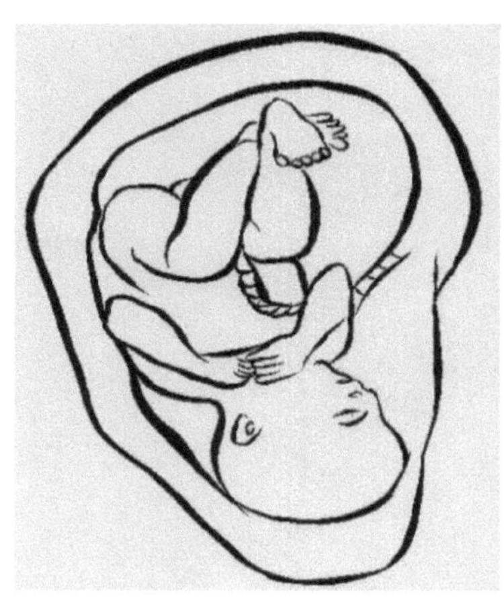

II. Auricular Points

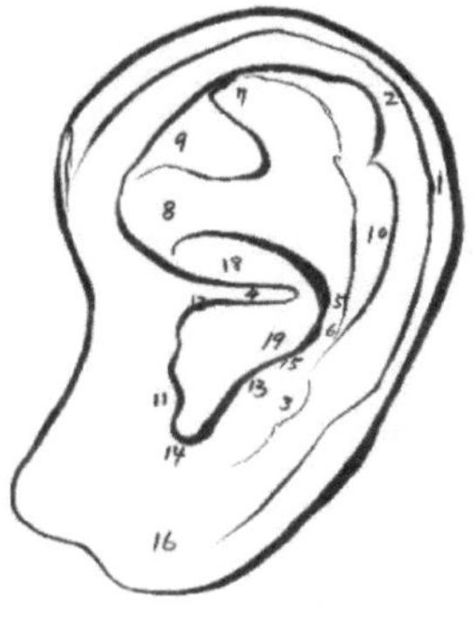

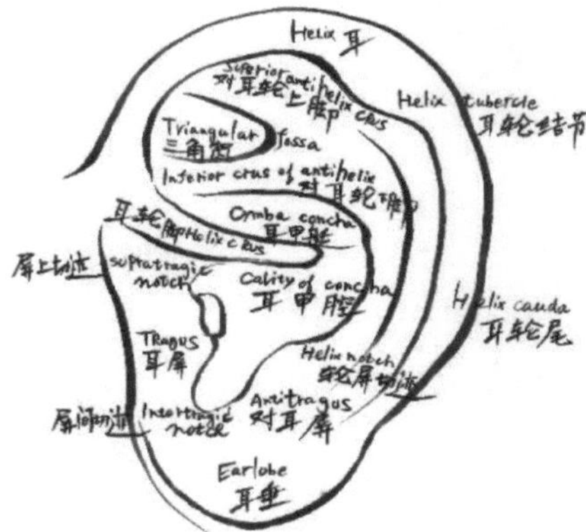

The anterior aspect

Auricular points are specific stimulating points on the ear. When the disorder occurs in the parts of the body, then it may appear various reactions at the corresponding areas of the ear. Thus, to make a diagnosis, it can be taken to stimulate the sensitive sites, and to prevent diseases.

1.The Corresponding Regional Anatomy of the Acupuncture Points

1.1. Distribution of Ear Points

The distribution of ear points on the ear follows a certain scheme.

The ear is compared to an inverted fetus with the head down towards the top. Ear points corresponding to head and face are near Earlobe. The points corresponding to the upper limbs are at the Scapha. Lower limbs are around the superior and inferior crus of Antihelix. Internal organs are Cymba Concha and Cavity of Concha.

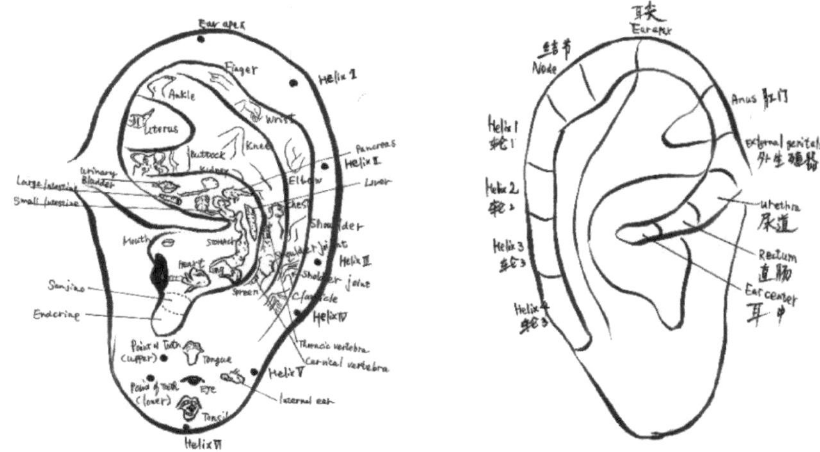

Ear Points for the corresponding regional anatomy   1. Points on the Helix

III. Auricular points Location, Function and Applicable Disease

1. Points on the Helix (Erlunxuewei 耳轮穴位)

1. Ear Center (Erzhong 耳中)

Location: On the Helix.
Function: Relax muscular spasm.
              Control Qi, Blood circulation and dispel wind and
              relieve pain.

Treatment: Hiccup, Vomiting, Blood deficiency/stasis/heat, hemorrhage, metrorrhagia.

2. Rectum (Zhichang 直肠)

Location: On the Helix.
Function: Laxation and alleviate diarrhea.
Treatment: Constipation, Diarrhea, prolapse anus, Hemorrhoid.

3. Urethra (Niaodao 尿道)

Location: On the Helix.
Function: Heat away and dampness. Relieve the muscular spasm and pain.
Treatment: Bed-wetting, frequent urination, painful urination, pruritis of the genitals.

4. External genitals (Waishengzhiqi 外生殖器)

Location: On the Helix.
Function: Clear heat and dampness in Liver and Gallbladder. Clear blood heat, dispel wind, relieve itching for sexual function.
Treatment: Various genitals diseases.
Testitis, vaginitis, itching vulvae.

5. Anus (Gangmen 肛门)

Location: On the Helix.
Function: Clear heat and relieve swelling and pain.
Promote laxation and blood flow.
Treatment: Prolapse anus, hemorrhoid.

6. Ear apex (Erjian 耳尖)

Location: On the top of the Helix.
Function: Clear heat and remove toxic substance.
              Calm liver, cool blood, relieve itching and swelling pain.
Treatment: Hypertension, fever, Eye disease, eczema, urticaria.

7. Node (Jiejie 结节)

Location: On the tubercle of the Helix.
Function: Clear heat and toxic in Liver.
              Relieve the depressed Liver and regulate the circulation of Qi.
Treatment: Hepatitis, Headache, dizziness.
              Pain around the waist and armpit of the body region.

8. Helix 1 (Lunyi1 轮 1)
9. Helix 2 (Lunyi2 轮 2)
10.Helix 3 (Lunyi3 轮 3)
11.Helix 4 (Lunyi4 轮 4)

Location: On the Helix.
Function: Clear heat and remove toxic substances.
              Treatment: Cold, respiratory tract infection, tonsillitis. Clear heat and various inflammation of syndrome.
Treatment: Cold, respiratory tract infection, tonsillitis. Clear heat and various inflammation of syndrome.

2. Points on the Scapha (Erzhou 耳舟)

1. Finger (Zhi 指)

Location: On the uppermost part of the Scaphoid fossa.
Function: Promote the blood circulation, dispel the wind, relieve pain and inflammation.
Treatment: Pain, numbness, sprain of the finger joint.

2. Wrist (Wan 腕)

Location: Inferior to the finger point.
Function: Promote the blood circulation, dispel the wind, relieve pain.
Treatment: Wrist pain sprain the wrist joint.

3. Wind stream (Fengxi 风溪)

Location: Between the finger point and wrist.
Function: Promote the blood flow, dispel the wind and itching, relieve cough and asthma.
Treatment: Asthma, allergic rhinitis and colitis, acne, urticaria, eczema.

4. Elbow (Zhou 肘)

Location: Inferior to the wrist point.
Function: Promote the blood flow. Dispel the wind. Relieve the pain.
Treatment: Elbow pain, tennis elbow, sprain elbow joint and rheumatic arthritis.

5. Shoulder (Jian 肩)

Location: Inferior to the elbow point.
Function: Promote the blood flow. Dispel the wind. Relieve the pain.

Treatment: Shoulder pain, sprain of shoulder joint, upper limbs dysfunction, pain by cervical spondylosis.

6. Clavicle (Suogu 锁骨)

Location: Inferior to the shoulder point.
Function: Dispel the wind, clear the dampness. Relieve the pain.
Treatment: Shoulder pain, back pain, neck pain, rheumatic pain, stiff neck.

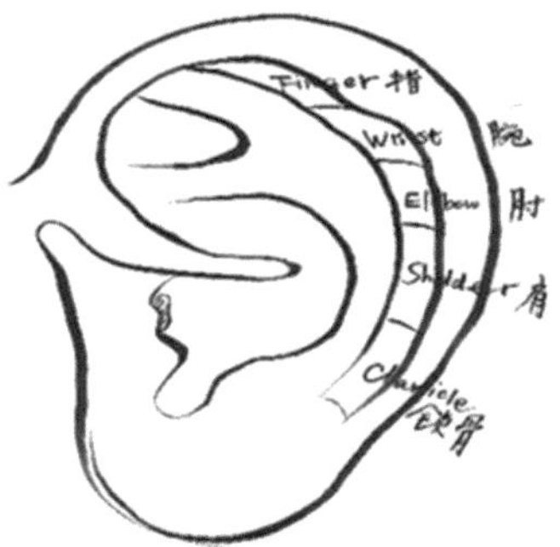

2. Points on the Scapha

3. Points on the Antihelix

3. Points on the Antihelix (Duierlunxuewei 对耳轮穴位)

1. Heel (Gen 跟)

Location: On the anterior and superior crus of the antihelix.
Function: Promote the blood flow, dispel the wind.
Strengthen the muscles and bones. Relieve the swelling and pain.
Treatment: Heel pain, injury swelling etc.

2. Toe (Zhi 趾)

Location: On the posterior and superior crus of the antihelix.
Function: Blood circulation, relieve pain.
Treatment: Arthritis, pain, pruritus of the toe joints.

3. Ankle (Huai 踝)

Location: On the upper one-third of the superior crus of the antihelix.
Function: Promote the blood flow, dispel the wind relieve the swelling and pain.
Treatment: Pain, dysfunction sprain of the ankle joint.

4. Knee (Xi 膝)

Location: On the middle one-third of the superior crus.
Function: Dispel the wind, clear the dampness and relieve pain.
Treatment: Swelling and pain of knee joint , rheumatic arthritis, sprain of the knee joint.

5. Hip (Kuan 髋)

Location: On the lower one-third of the superior crus of the antihelix.
Function: Promote the blood flow, dispel the wind relieve pain.
Treatment: Sciatic nerve, lumbosacral pain, arthritis.

6. Sciatic nerv (Zuogushenjing 坐骨神经)

Location: On the anterior two-thirds of the inferior crus.
Function: Strengthen the muscles and bones, relieve pain.
Treatment: Sciatica, paralysis of the lower limbs.

7. Sympathesis (Jiaogan 交感)

Location: Crus of the antihelix and the internal edge of the Helix.
Function: Relax of the spasm of the muscle. Treat the visceral pain.
Treatment: Insomnia, hyperhidrosis neurosis of visceral organs, asthma, gastric ulcer, visceral colic.

8. Gluteus (Tun 臀)

Location: On the posterior one-third of the inferior crus.
Function: Promote the blood flow, dispel the wind, relieve pain.
Treatment: Sciatica, buttocks and sacral pain.

9. Abdomen (Fu 腹)

Location: On the anterior and superior two-fifths of the antihelix.
Function: Muscular spasm relieve pain.
Treatment: Abdominal pain and distension, diarrhea, constipation, lumbar sprain,
gallstone, dysmenorrhea, irregular menstruation.

10. Lumbosacral vertebrae (Yaodizhui 腰骶椎)

Location: On the posterior of the abdomen.
Function: Promote the blood flow, relieve pain.
Strengthen the bone. Reinforce bone.
Treatment: Lumbosacral pain, dysfunction of lower limbs, lumber muscle strain, numbness of lower limbs, rheumatoid arthritis. Urinary incontinence, sciatica.

11.Chest (Xiong 胸)

Location: On middle and anterior two-fifths of the antihelix.
Function: Regulate Qi and alleviate depression.
Treatment: Heart disease, Zoster, costal chondritis, intercostal neuralgia.

12.Thoracic vertebrae (Xiongzhui 胸椎)

Location: Posterior to the chest point.
Function: Promote the blood flow, dispel the wind, relieve pain.
Treatment: Chest and back pain, back muscles strain, intercostal neuralgia.

13.Neck (Jing 颈)

Location: On the anterior and inferior one-fifth of the antihelix.
Function: Regulate thyroid function.
Treatment: Stiff neck, cervical sprain, thyroid swelling, hyperthyroidism.

14.Cervical vertebrae (Jingzhui 颈椎)

Location: Posterior to the neck point.
Function: Promote the blood flow, dispel wind, strengthen the muscles and bones, relieve the pain.
Treatment: Stiff neck, rheumatoid arthritis, paralysis of the upper limbs, itching, thyroid enlargement.

4. Points on the Triangular Fossa (sanjiaowoxuewei 三角窝穴位)

1. Superior triangular fossa (Jiaowoshang 角窝上)

Location: On the anterior and superior one-third of triangular fossa.
Function: Decrease the blood pressure, regulate and nourish the Liver and Kidney, nourish the blood.
Treatment: Hypertension, headache, vertigo.

2. Internal genitals (Neishengzhiqi 内生殖器)

Location: On the anterior and inferior one-third of the triangular fossa.

Function: Regulate menstruation, nourish Kidney, pelvic infection.

Treatment: Irregular menstruation, dysmenorrhea, pelvic inflammation, impotence prostatitis, male and female infertility.

3. Middle triangular fossa (Jiaowozhong 角窝中)

Location: On the middle one-third of the triangular fossa.

Function: Alleviate depression, regulate Qi.

Treatment: Bronchial asthma, fullness of the chest, shortness of breath.

4. Shenmen (神门)

Location: On the posterior and superior one-third of the triangular fossa.

Function: Relieve muscular spasm, pain, and inflammation. Calm Liver.

Treatment: (1) Hypertension.
(2) urticaria, eczema, cough.
(3) headache, inflammation.

5. Pelvis (Penqiang 盆腔)

Location: On the posterior and inferior one-third of the triangular fossa.

Function: Clear heat and dampness. Relieve pain.

Treatment: Pelvic inflammation, prostatitis, irregular menstruation, lower limb pain, abdominal pain.

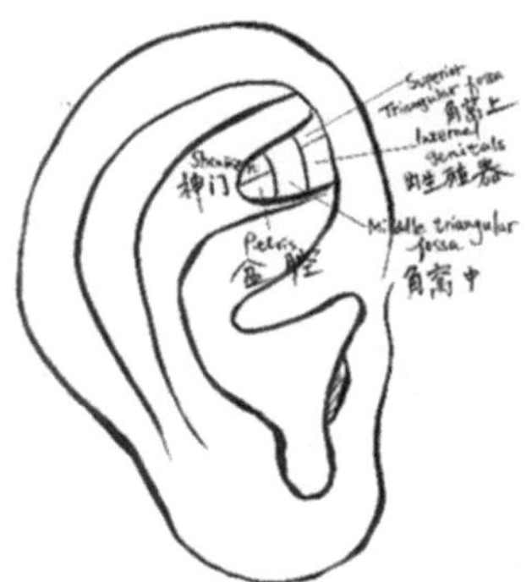

4. Points on the Triangular Fossa   **5. Points on the Tragus**

5. Points on the Tragus (Erpingxuewei 耳屏穴位)

1. External ear (Waier 外耳)

Location: On the upper edge of the tragus.
Function: Promote blood circulation, clear the blood stasis, calm down and relieve pain.
Treatment: Dizziness, migraine, deafness and tinnitus, cervical pain.

2. Apex of the tragus (Pingjian 屏尖)

Location: On the posterior edge of the tragus.
Function: Anti-inflammation, reduce fever, tranquil pain.
Treatment: Toothache, Fever, inflammation, pain.

3. External nose (Waibi 外鼻)

Location: The center of the external edge of the tragus.
Function: Clear heat, promote the blood flow, relieve pain.

Treatment: Rhinitis, nasal obstruction.

4. Adrenal gland (Shenshangxian 肾上腺)

Location: On the apex of the inferior tragus.

Function: Anti-infection relieves cough and asthma, anti-rheumatism, coordinate the function of adrenal gland.

Treatment: (1) Rheumatic arthritis.

(2) Allergic disease, asthma, cough, inflammations.

(3) Hemorrhagic disease, hypotension.

5. Pharynx and larynx (Yanhou 咽喉)

Location: On the superior of the internal side of the tragus.

Function: Expel toxin, relieve inflammation and swelling, resolve sputum and clear the throat.

Treatment: Pharyngitis, tonsillitis, hoarseness, bronchitis, bronchial asthma.

6. Internal nose (Neibi 内鼻)

Location: On the inferior half of the internal of the tragus.

Function: Dispel wind, stop bleeding.

Treatment: Cold, nasal obstruction, rhinitis, epistaxis.

7. Anterior intertragal notch (Pingjianqian 屏间前)

Location: On the lowest part of the tragus, on the inferior edge of the tragus.

Function: Clear heat, promote blood circulation, clear the heat in brain for brightening eyes.

Treatment: Dizziness, headache, glaucoma, myopia, retinitis.

6. Points on the Antitragus (Duierpingxuewei 对耳屏穴位)

1. Forehead (E 额)

Location: On the anterior part of the antitragus.
Function: Strengthen the function of brain and brighten eyes.
Treatment: Dizziness, insomnia, myopia, sinusitis, rhinitis.

2. Posterior intertragal notch (Pingjianhou 屏间后)

Location: Posterior to the notch between tragus and antitragus, on the inferior edge of the antitragus.
Function: Relieve the heat and toxin, cool the blood, brighten the eyes.
Treatment: Glaucoma, stye, eye disease.

3. Temple (Nie 颞)

Location: On the middle of the external side of the antitragus.
Function: Regulate Qi, relieve Liver and Gallbladder, brighten eye, relieve tinnitus.
Treatment: Dizziness, migraine, tinnitus.

4. Occiput (Zhen 枕)

Location: On the posterior of the external side of the antitragus.
Function: Clear heat, dispel itching, relieve cough and asthma, brighten eyes.
Treatment: (1) Dizziness, headache, seasickness.
             (2) Meningitis, brain trauma,
             (3) Insomnia.

(4) Asthma.

5. Subcortex (Pizhixia 皮质下)

Location: On the medial side of the antitragus.
Function: dispel pain, relieve hiccup and vomiting, nourish the brain and calm the mind.
Treatment: (1) Gastritis, nausea, vomiting, abdominal distension, constipation, hiccup.
(2) Insomnia, dreaminess.

6. Apex of the antitragus (Duipingjian 对屏尖)

Location: On the apex of antitragus.
Function: Relieve cough and asthma, dispel itching.
Treatment: Cough, asthma, short breath, pruritus.

7. Central rim (Yuanzhong 缘中)

Location: On the antitragus, junction among the antitragus.
Function: Relieve muscular spasm, nourish the brain.
Treatment: Vertigo, cerebral concussion.

8. Brain stem (Naogan 脑干)

Location: On the antitragus, between antitragus and antihelix.
Function: Relieve muscular spasm, replenish the brain.
Treatment: Epilepsy, schizophrenia, neurosis, vertigo, headache.

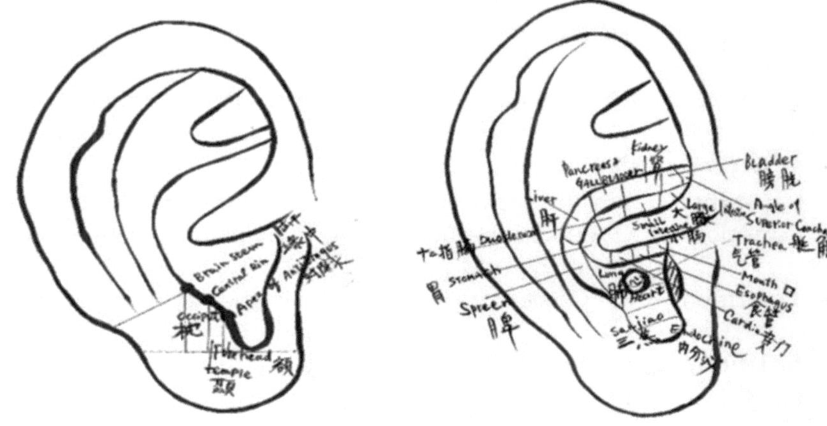

6.Points on the Antitragus	**7. Points on the Concha**

7. Points on the Concha (Erjiaxuewei 耳甲穴位)

1. Mouth (Kou 口)

Location: On the anterior one-third of the concha, under the inferior crus of the antihelix.

Function: Relieve muscular spasm, cough, asthma and pain. Regulate gastrointestinal function.

Treatment: Bronchial asthma, cough, insomnia, oral ulcer, facial paralysis.

2. Esophagus (Shidao 食道)

Location: On the middle one-third of the concha.

Function: Treat dysphagia, promote appetite, regulate esophagus.

Treatment: Chest distress, short breath, difficult to fall asleep.

3. Cardia (Penmen 喷门)

272

Location: On the anterior one-third of the concha.
Function: Relieve spasm, regulate stomach, promote appetite.
Treatment: Nausea, cardio spasm, vomiting, chest discomfort.

4. Stomach (Wei 胃)

Location: On the terminus of the superior crus of the helix.
Function: Regulate the flow of Qi, invigorate Spleen, relieve vomiting and pain.
Treatment   (1) Gastric ulcer gastrointestinal dysfunction.

5. Duoderum (Shierzhichang 十二指肠)

Location: On the posterior one-third of the inferior crus of the helix.
Function: Relieve spasm and pain, regulate gastrointestinal function.
Treatment: Abdominal distension, diarrhea, cholecystitis.

6. Small intestine (Xiaochang 小肠)

Location: On the middle one-third of the superior crus of the helix.
Function: Clear dampness and heat, relieve diarrhea, promote circulation of Qi and remove obstruction. Eliminate heat.
Treatment: Diarrhea, abdominal distension, intestinal tuberculosis.

7. Large intestine (Dachang 大肠)

Location: On the anterior one-third of the inferior crus.
Function: Remove heat, relieve cough, diarrhea.
Treatment: Diarrhea, intestinal dysfunction. Cough asthma, cold pneumonia respiratory tract disease, acne.

8. Appendix (Lanwei 阑尾)

Location: Between the point of Large intestine and Small intestine.

Function: Clear heat, promote blood circulation.

Treatment: Diarrhea. Appendicitis.

9. Angle of superior concha (Tingjiao 艇角)

Location: On the anterior of the concha, inferior to the inferior crus.

Function: Nourish Kidney, eliminate dampness, promote blood circulation, eliminate stagnation and remove abdominal mass.

Treatment: Bronchial asthma, Epistaxis.

10. Bladder (Pangguang 膀胱)

Location: On the middle of the concha inferior to the inferior crus of the helix.

Function: Relieve heat and dampness, regulate Qi circulation, relieve pain.

Treatment: Backache, spinal column pain, sciatica.

11. Kidney (Shen 肾)

Location: On the posterior of the concha inferior to the inferior crus of the helix.

Function: Nourish Yin and strengthen Yang of Kidney, strengthen the back, improve eyesight.

Treatment: Heel and leg pain, dizziness, insomnia, brain and spinal marrow, rheumatoid arthritis.

12. Ureter (Shuniaoguan 输尿管)

Location: Between Kidney and Bladder.

Function: Clear heat and dampness in lower Jiao, relax spasm.
Treatment: Urinary infections.

13. Pancreas and gallbladder (Yidan 胰胆)

Location: On the posterior and superior of the superior concha.
Function: Disperse the depressed Qi of Liver and Gallbladder. Relieve pain.
Treatment: (1) Cholecystitis, fullness of hypochondriac region.
(2) Diabetes mellitus, insomnia, tinnitus, migræne.

14. Liver (Gan 肝)

Location: On the posterior and inferior part.
Function: Smooth Liver, Qi and blood circulation, remove blood stasis.
Treatment: (1) Hepatitis.
(2) Dysfunctional menstruation, dysmenorrhea, dizziness, gynecologic diseases.
(3) Muscle spasm, limb numbness convulsion of hand and foot

15. Center of superior concha (Tingzhong 艇中)

Location: Between the Small Intestine and Kidney.

Function: Regulate of Qi circulation, relieve pain.
Treatment: Abdominal pain and distension.

16. Spleen (Pi 脾)

Location: On the posterior and superior of the inferior concha.

Function: Clear dampness and heat, raise Qi, function of digestion and transportation.
Treatment: Edema, stagnation of phlegm and dampness, hemorrhagic syndrome, metrorrhagia, metrostaxis, uterine bleeding.

17. Heart (Xin 心)

Location: On the central and the inferior concha.
Function: Eliminate heart-fire, clear blood stasis
Treatment: (1) Heart disease, neurosis, insomnia, dreaminess, night sweating.
(2) hoarseness, pharyngitis.
(3) Skin diseases.

18. Trachea (Qiguan 气管)

Location: Locates side of heart.
Function: Relieve cough and sputum, asthma and sore throat. Expel wind.
Treatment: Bronchial asthma, cold, cough, pharyngitis.

19. Lung (Fei 肺)

Location: Around the heart and trachea.
Function: Promote Qi circulation. Eliminate wind and itching. Relieve cough, asthma.
Treatment: Respiratory diseases, bronchitis, bronchial asthma, palpitation, short breath, oppressed feeling in chest, cough.

20. Sanjiao (三焦)

Location: Posterior and inferior to the canal, between Lung and Endocrine point.

Function: Coordinate the function of Zang Fu organs, Qi circulation, regulate spleen, nourish heart and lung, invigorate kidney.

Treatment: (1) Coronary heart disease, hypochondriac pain short breath.
(2) Edema
(3) Tinnitus, deafness
(4) Pain of the lateral side of the upper limbs.

21. Endocrine (Neifenmi 内分泌)

Location: Inside the notch between the tragus and antitragus.

Function: Anti-infection, promote the blood flow, relieve dampness.

Treatment: Dysmenorrhea, menopausal syndrome, obesity, irregular menstruation, hyperthyroidism.

8. Points on the Earlobe (Erchuixuewei 耳垂穴位)

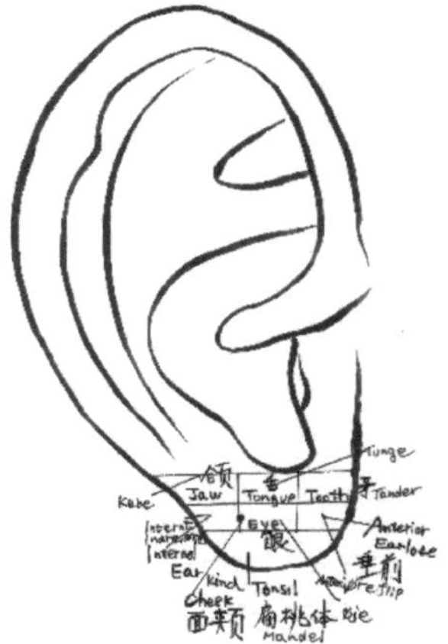

1. Teeth (Ya 牙)

Location: On the anterior and superior of the earlobe.
Function: Clear the heat, relieve pain.
Treatment: Hypotension.

2. Tongue (She 舌)

Location: On the middle and superior of the earlobe.
Function: Clear the heat in the heart, promote the blood flow.
Treatment: Split tongue, ulcer.

3. Jaw (He 颌)

Location: On the posterior and superior of the ear lobe.
Function: Dispel wind, relieve pain.
Treatment: Toothache, arthritis.

4. Anterior earlobe (Chuiqian 垂前)

Location: On the anterior and middle of the earlobe.
Function: Inhibit of brain cortex, relieve pain.
Treatment: Dizziness, insomnia, dreaminess, palpitation.

5. Eye (Yan 眼)

Location: On the center of the earlobe.
Function: Clear heat. Smooth Qi circulation in liver and bright eyes.
Treatment: Conjunctivitis, glaucoma, cataract, myopia, optic atrophy.

6. Internal ear (Neier 内耳)

Location: On the posterior and middle portion of the earlobe.
Function: Dispel wind and heat, improve the function of hearing.
Treatment: Deafness, tinnitus.

7. Cheek (Mianjia 面颊)

Location: Between the eye and internal ear.
Function: Dispel the wind, the spasm. Relieve swelling.
Treatment: Bell's palsy, acne, facial wrinkles.

8. Tonsil (Biantaoti 扁桃体)

Location: On the inferior portion of the earlobe.
Function: Clear heat and toxin, anti-inflammation, relieve swelling.
Treatment: Tonsillitis, pharyngitis.

9. Points on the Posterior Surface of the Auricle (Erbeixuewei 耳背穴位)

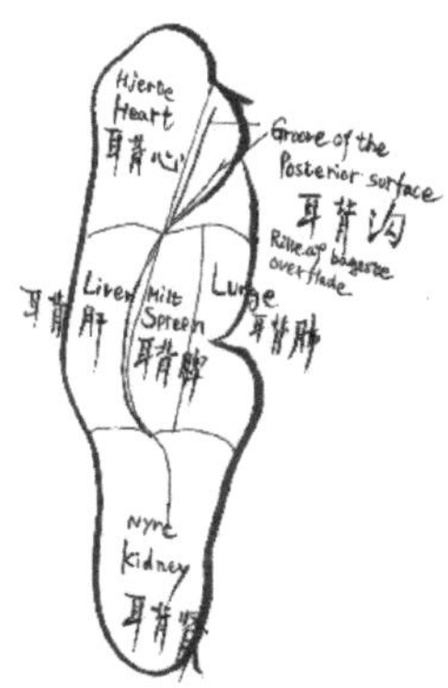

9. Posterior Surface

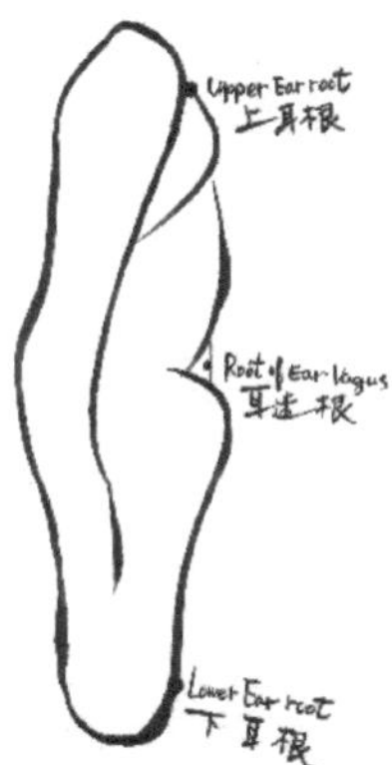

10. Ear Root

1. Heart of the posterior surface (Erbeixin 耳背心)

Location: On the superior, the posterior.
Function: Clear Heart heat, relieve mental stress.

Treatment: Hypertension, palpitation, insomnia, headache.

2. Lung of the posterior surface (Erbeifei 耳背肺)
Location: On the middle, internal, posterior. surface.
Function: Relieve cough, the flow of Lung Qi, relieve asthma.
Treatment: Bronchitis, bronchial asthma, cutaneous pruritus.

3. Spleen of the posterior surface (Erbeipi 耳背脾)
Location: On the center of the posterior surface.
Function: Regulate Spleen and Stomach, relieve pain and digestion.
Treatment: Gastritis, stomachache, poor appetite.

4. Liver of the posterior surface (Erbeigan 耳背肝)

Location: On the middle and external part of the posterior.
Function: Relieve Liver and Gallbladder, Qi circulation.
Treatment: Pain of hypochondriac region, cholecystitis.

5. Kidney of the posterior surface (Erbeishen 耳背肾)
Location: On the inferior part of the posterior.
Function: Nourish Liver and Kidney, strengthen bone and invigorate marrow, relieve spasm.

6. Groove of the posterior surface (Erbeigou 耳背沟)
Location: The groove formed by antihelix, superior, inferior antihelix, and on the posterior.
Function: Calm Liver, dispel wind, decrease blood pressure, relieve itching.
Treatment: Hypertension, headache.

10.Points on the Ear Root (Ergenxuewei 耳根穴位)

1. Upper ear root (Shangergen 上耳根)

Location: On the uppermost part.
Function: Clear blood-heat.
Treatment: Epistaxis, paralysis.

2. Root of ear vagus (Ermigen 耳迷根)

Location: In the posterior groove formed by Helix.
Function: Clear heat and dampness, relieve spasm.
Treatment: Abdominal pain, diarrhea, headache, insomnia, dizziness, stomachache, hypertension, retention of urine.

3. Lower ear root (Xiaergen 下耳根)

Location: On the lowest part.
Function: Nourish Liver and Kidney, relieve mental stress.
Treatment: Hypotension, Bell's palsy.

CHARPTER 5 Acupuncture Needling Techniques

1. Manipulation of the Needle

(1) The Needles and how to use them

- **The filiform needle:**
  is widely used and flexible. It is better to start practicing with a shorter and thicker needle for the beginners.

- **Practice with sheets of paper:**
  Fold fine soft tissue into a small packet about 5 x 8 cm in size and 1 cm thick, and then puncture it. Hold the paper packet in the left hand and the handle of the needle with the thumb, index and middle fingers of the right hand. Rotate the needle in and out. As your finger force grows stronger, the thickness of the packet may be increased.

- **Practice with a small cotton cushion:**
  Cotton cushion of about 5-6 cm. in diameter wrapped in gauze. Hold the cushion with the left hand and the needle with the thumb, index and middle fingers of the right hand. Insert the needle into it and practice the lift-thrust and rotation procedure.

- **Practice on your body:**
  This may follow the manipulation methods on paper packet and cotton cushion, so as to have personal experience of the acupuncture sensation in clinical practice.

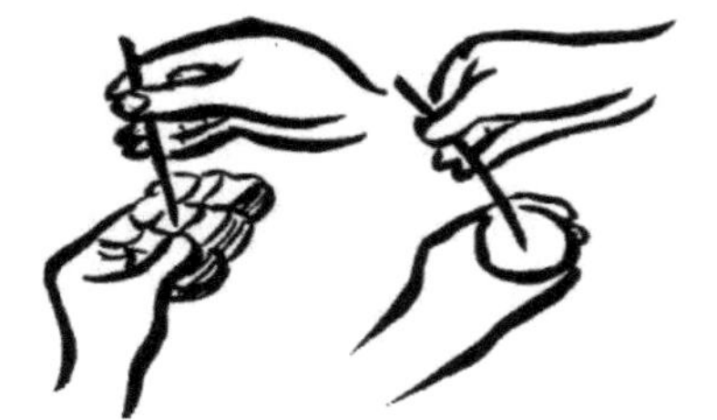

with sheets of paper   with a small cushion

(2) The Angle of Needle Insertion

Angle: There are generally three angles for insertion.

- Perpendicular: the needle is inserted perpendicularly forming a 90-degree angle with the skin surface.
- Oblique: The needle is inserted obliquely to form an angle of 45 degrees with the skin surface.
- Transverse: The needle is inserted transversely to form an angle of 15 degrees with the skin surface.

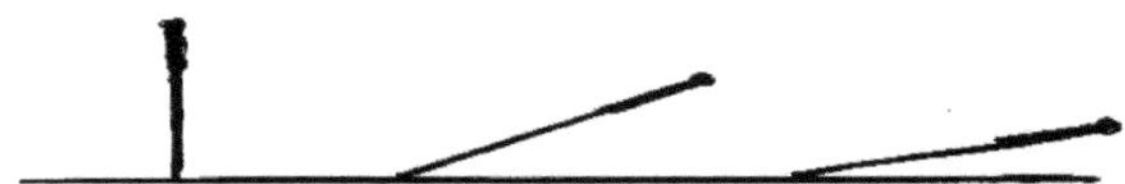

(3) Depth of Needle Insertion

It depends on the thickness of the tissue where the point is located and pathological condition. As a rule, points on the extremities, abdomen and lumbosacral region may be punctured deeper than others.

(4) Insertion of the Needle

Generally, the needle is held with the right hand, with the thumb and index fingers holding the handle of the needle and the middle finger backing the index finger near the needle root. The left hand, the pressing hand, presses upon the area close to the point. The coordination of the two hands is conductive to the swift penetration of the needle tip into the skin, which reduces pain on insertion.

According to the length of the needle and the location of the point, there are various methods of insertion.

The Main Insertion techniques:

- **Inserting the needle aided by the pressure of the finger of the pressing hand:**
  Press beside the acupuncture point with the nail of the thumb or the index finger of the pressing hand, then insert the needle into the point against the nail. The method is suitable for puncturing with short needles such as for needing PC-6(Neiguan 内关), KI-6 (Zhaohai 照海), BL-60 (Kunlun 昆仑) etc.

- **Inserting the needle with the help of the puncturing and pressing hands:**
  Hold the tip of the needle with the thumb and index fingers of the left hand, leaving 0.2-0.3 cm. of its tip exposed, and hold the needle handle with the thumb and index finger of the right hand. As the needle tip is directly over the selected point, insert the needle swiftly into the skin with the left hand, meanwhile the right hand presses the needle downward to the required depth. This method is suitable for puncturing with long needles, such as those used in puncturing, GB-30 (Huantiao 环跳), BL-54 (Zhibian 秩边) etc.

- **Inserting the needle with the fingers stretching the skin:**
  Stretch the skin where the point is located to cause tension with the thumb and the index finger of the pressing hand to facilitate the insertion of the needle. This method is indicated for points where the skin is loosed such as ST-25 (Tianshu 天枢), Ren-4 (Guanyuan 关元) etc. on the abdomen.

- **Inserting the needle by pinching up the skin:**
  Pinch up the skin at the point with the thumb and index finger of the pressing hand, insert the needle into the skin sidewise with the right hand. This method is suitable for puncturing points of the head and face where the muscle and skin are thin, such as BL-2 (Zanzhu 攒竹), ST-4 (Dicang 地仓), EX-HN3 (Yintang 印堂) etc.

(5) Withdrawal of the Needle

To prevent the bleeding at the site of puncture and the after sensation, it is necessary to rotate the needle back and forth gently before withdrawing it, then press the puncture site gently with cotton ball stick upon withdrawal.

(6) Precaution

- It is advisable to apply few needles or to delay giving acupuncture treatment for patients who are over fatigued and very weak.
- It is contraindicated to puncture points on the lower abdomen and lumbosacral region for women pregnant under three months. After three months of pregnancy it is also contraindicated to puncture the points of the upper abdomen, and those causing strong sensation

such as LI-4 (Hegu 合谷), SP-6 (Sanyinjiao 三阴交), BL-60 (Kunlun 昆仑), BL-67 (Zhiyin 至阴). The fontanelle of infants should not be punctured.

2. Plum Blossom Needle

It is a needling method of treatment by using several small needles to tap on the skin of the corresponding area shallowly. This superficial tapping is particularly suitable to treat disorders of the nervous system and skin diseases.

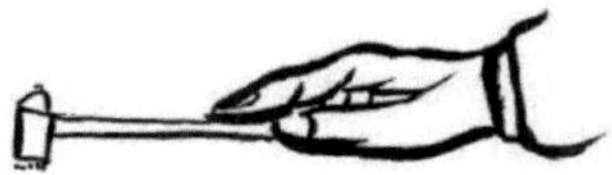

Indications:
It is applicable to hypertension, headache, dizziness, vertigo, insomnia, pain of back and loin, numbness, painful joints, paralysis, myopia, dysmenorrhea, loose hair.

Manipulation:
After routine and local sterilization, hold the handle of the needle and tap vertically on the skin surface with a flexible movement of the wrist. The tapping may be light or slight until the skin becomes congested, or slight bleeding appears.

The area to be tapped may be along the course of the meridians, or on the affected area.

Precautions:
Tapping should avoid applying to the local trauma and ulcers. After tapping, the local skin surface should be cleaned and sterilized to prevent infection.

3. Electro Acupuncture

It is a kind of therapy by which the needle is attached to a trace pulse current after it is inserted to the selected acupoint for the purpose of producing synthetic effect of electric and needling stimulation. They generate low-frequency impulse current which is close to bioelectric current in the human body.

Manipulations

After the needle is inserted into a certain acupoint and the needling sensation is felt, adjust the output potential instrument of the electro-acupuncture stimulator to zero, then connect the two output wires with the two needle handles, select the required waveform and frequency, and then gradually amplify the output current to the tolerance of the patient. After a few minutes, the human body will be adaptive to the stimulation and feel that the stimulation is getting weaker. At the time, increase the output current appropriately. The stimulation continues for 10-20 min. or longer according to the pathological conditions of the patient. When the treatment is finished, the output potential instrument is adjusted back to zero.

Precautions:

Before using the electro-acupuncture apparat, it needs to examine in good condition and that the switches are off.
The current should be reinforced gradually in adjustment. Sudden increase should be avoided. The patient can hold the apparat and use the switches in suitable channel.

4. Scalp Acupuncture

Scalp acupuncture is a therapy with which specific zone on the head are punctured to prevent or treat diseases.

4.1 Location of Stimulating zone and Indication

There are two standard lines that are used to divide the stimulation areas.

- Anterior-Posterior Midline:
  The midline connecting the midpoint between the eyebrows (the anterior point of the midline) to the inferior border of the external occipital protuberance (the posterior point of the midline).
- The Eyebrow-Occiput Line:
  The line connecting the midpoint of the superior border of the eyebrow to the tip of the external occipital protuberance.

(1) Motor Zone

- Location: The superior point is located 0.5 cm posterior to the midpoint of the anterior-posterior midline as the upper point, the inferior point at the junction of the brow-occipital line and the anterior border of temporal hairline as the lower point. The line connecting between these two points is the motor zone.
- Indications: The line is divided into five equal parts. The upper 1/5 is the motor zone of the lower limb paralysis; the middle 2/5 for upper limb paralysis; lower 2/5 for central facial paralysis, motor aphasia, salvation, dysphonia, etc.

(2) Sensory Zone

- Location: The horizontal line 1.5 cm posterior to the motor zone. It is divided into five equal parts. The upper 1/5 for lower limb, middle 2/5 for upper limb, and lower 2/5 for head and face.
- Indications: The upper 1/5 for contralateral lumbocrural pain, numbness, occiput pain, neck pain vertigo, tinnitus. The middle 2/5 for contralateral upper

limb pain, numbness, paresthesia. The low 2/5 for contralateral facial numbness, migraine temporomandibular arthritis.

(3) **Control Zone of Chorea and Tremor**

- Location: The horizontal line 1.5 cm anterior to the motor zone.
- Indications: Chorea, Parkinson's disease, etc.

(4) **Vertigo-Auditory Zone**

- Location: This area is a 4 cm. The horizontal line 1.5 cm directly from above the auricular apex.
- Indications: Tinnitus, loss of hearing, vertigo, hypoacusis.

(5) **the 2nd Speech Zone**

- Location: This area is a 3 cm. The straight line 2 cm posterior and inferior to the parietal tubercule and parallel to the anteroposterior midline, stretching 3 cm straightly and downwards.
- Indications: Nominal aphasia.

(6) **The 3rd Speech Zone**

- Location: 4 cm horizontal line from the midpoint of the vertigo and hearing zone.
- Indications: Sensory aphasia.

(7) **Applying Zone**

- Location: Take the parietal tubercles a starting point, and draw a vertical line from this point, at the same time draw the other two lines from the point separately forwards and backwards, at line 40° angle with the vertical line, each of the three lines is 3 cm in length.

- Indications: Apraxia.

(8) The Foot Motor Sensory Zone
- Location: Two straight lines 3 cm stretching back 1cm from both sides of the midpoint of the antero-posterior midline and parallel to the midline.
- Indications: Paralysis, pain and numbness, acute lumbar sprain, nocturia, cerebro-cortical polyuria.

(9) Visual Zone
- Location: 4 cm straight line upwards 1cm from both sides of the posterior point of the anteroposterior midline and parallel to the midline.
- Indications: Cerebro-cortical visual disturbance.

(10) Balance Zone
- Location: 4cm straight line downwards and 3.5 cm from both sides of the antero-posterior midline and parallel to the midline.
- Indications: Equilibrium disturbance caused by cerebellum disease.

(11) Stomach Zone
- Location: Straight line 2 cm stretching upwards from the hair line directly over the pupil and parallel to the midline.
- Indications: Gastric pain, epigastric discomfort.

(12) Thoracic Cavity Zone
- Location: Between the stomach zone and antero-posterior midline 2 straight lines 2 cm stretching from the hairline upwards and downwards respectively and parallel to the midline.
- Indications: Asthma, chest pain, palpitation, hiccup, coronary artery insufficiency.

(13) Reproduction Zone
- Location: 2 cm straight line from the frontal angle and parallel to the anterio-posterior midline.
- Indications: Dysfunctional uterine bleeding, pelvic inflammation, leukorrhagia, prolapse of uterus.

References 参考文献

1. Ding Xiaohong, Acupuncture- Moxibustion, 1999
2. Want Lingli, Chinese Acupuncture and Moxibustion, 2002
3. Zhang Yujuan, Practical Handbook on Acupuncture and Moxibustion, 1989
4. Geng Junying, Su Zhihong, Acupuncture and Moxibustion, 1997
5. Yu Changzheng, therapeutics of Acupuncture and Moxibustion, 1990
6. Deng Liangyue, Chinese Acupuncture and Moxibustion, 2008
7. Yan Jie, Skills with Illustrations of Chinese Acupuncture and Moxibustion, 1991
8. Sumiko Knudsen, Ear Acupuncture, 2020
9. Sumiko Knudsen, Body Acupuncture, Clinical Treatment, 2021

Other library of Traditional Chinese Medicine by Sumiko Knudsen

1. Acupuncture for Weight Loss
2. Acupuncture Meridians and Points
3. Ear Acupuncture
4. Body Acupuncture, Clinical Treatment